# The Herbal Remedies & Natural Medicine Bible

# 10 in 1

## The Ultimate Collection of Healing Herbs and Plants for Creating Natural Remedies, Infusions, Essential Oils, Tea, Tinctures & Antibiotics

By

Isabella Greene

# Table of Content

# SCAN THE QR CODE TO RECEIVE FREE 3 AMAZING TOOLS!

**The Herbal Harvest Logbook:** This tool will help you keep track of the herbs you gather or cultivate. Record vital information such as the harvest date, location, weather conditions, and more. Maintain a detailed record to maximize the effectiveness of your herbal practices.

**The Remedy Preparation Planner:** The remedy preparation planner will guide you through the process of creating herbal remedies. Organize your recipes, measurements, and instructions in one place, simplifying the production of natural remedies for personal well-being.

**Medicinal Plants Book:** Unlock the ancient wisdom of herbal healing with this comprehensive guide. Dive into the world of natural remedies and explore the therapeutic potential of another 55 potent medicinal plants.

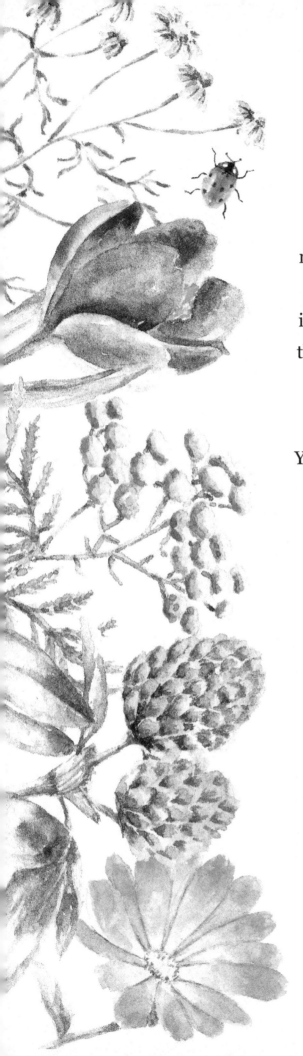

Dear Reader,

I trust my book on herbal remedies and natural medicine has been a helpful resource for your journey towards wellness. Your insights matter greatly to me. If you've found the information and remedies beneficial, or if there are areas that stood out, I would be grateful to hear your thoughts.

Your feedback is a compass for me to enhance future editions and works. Your experience can make a real difference for others exploring herbal remedies and natural medicine.

With gratitude,

Isabella Greene

# INTRODUCTION

Welcome to the fascinating world of natural therapies and botanical remedies. This book set invites you to journey through time, uncovering the old and the new secrets of plant-based healing passed down over generations. Our mission is to equip you with the tools and knowledge necessary to enhance your health naturally, seamlessly blending age-old herbal practices with evidence-backed research.

In today's fast-moving era, many of us gravitate towards non-conventional means to better our health and overall well-being. We're on a quest for remedies that are not just effective but also resonate with nature's rhythm. Herbal medicine stands out, emphasizing a whole-person approach, leveraging the healing prowess of plants to augment our body's inherent healing mechanisms.

"The Herbal Remedies & Natural Medicine Bible" collates insights and methods from diverse healing cultures. Think of it as your dependable companion towards optimal health. Whether you're an herbal aficionado or a newcomer to botanical cures, this set brings a treasure trove of information, inspiration, and hands-on advice to enrich your journey. No matter your familiarity, these pages promise to enhance your understanding of nature's pharmacy.

The inaugural book in this collection is a detailed guide to natural healing. It covers the nuances of herbalism, from plant recognition and ethical harvesting to the making and administering of herbal solutions. Dive deep into the myriad medicinal plants and discover their myriad uses, from soothing common ailments to fostering overall wellness.

We also touch upon areas like nutrition, aromatherapy, homeopathy, and the holistic art of mindfulness, highlighting the synergy of our physical, psychological, and emotional states. Benefit from actionable insights on integrating these organic approaches into your daily routines.

Safety and informed choices underscore our discussions throughout this collection. While nature's remedies can be immensely beneficial, partnering with healthcare professionals and being attuned to your body's needs is paramount. We urge readers to seek expert advice when faced with specific health challenges or when on prescribed medications.

Our ambition behind "The Herbal Remedies & Natural Medicine Bible" is to present an all-encompassing guide that allows you to champion your health holistically. Immerse yourself in the transformative magic of herbs, respect time-tested healing traditions, and stay abreast of current scientific breakthroughs.

As you navigate the path to wellness, let this book collection be both your mentor and muse. Envision it as a blueprint leading you to a life of equilibrium, vitality, and harmony. By the end, we trust you'll be equipped with the insights and self-assuredness to harness nature's restorative essence, awakening your body's utmost health potential.

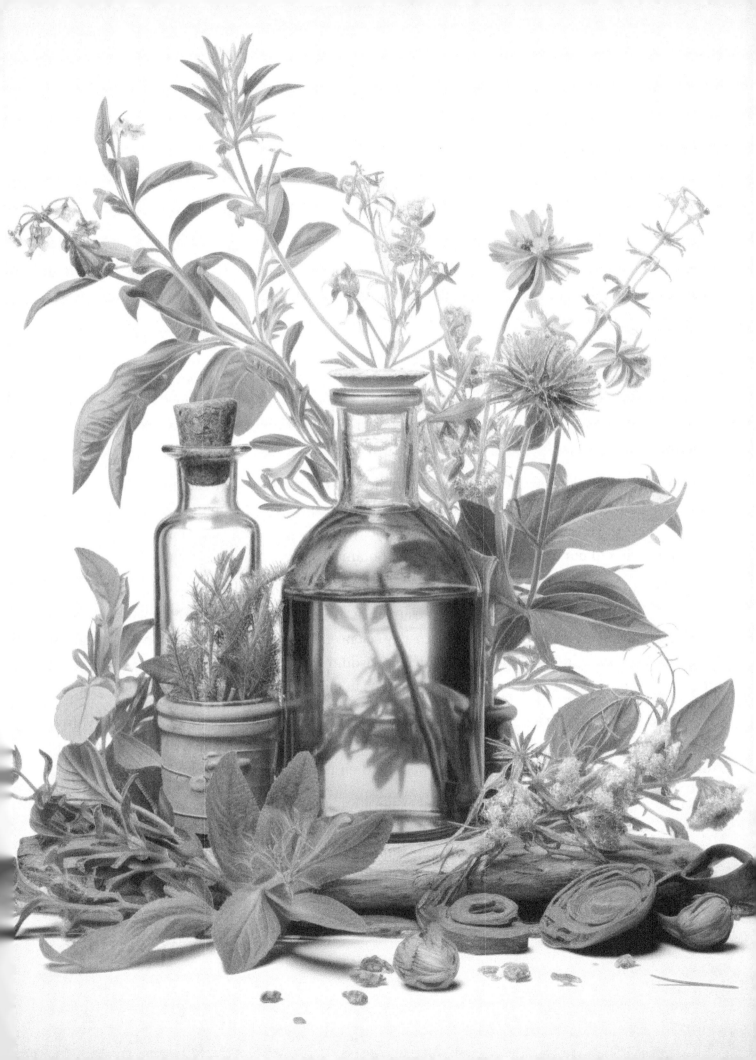

# BOOK 1: HISTORY AND INTRODUCTION OF HERBALISM

## Introduction

From the outset of human history, nature has been our foremost healer, providing remedies that nurture our well-being and health. Herbalism, the timeless practice of utilizing plants for their healing properties, stands as a testament to humanity's bond with the rhythms of the natural world. Welcome to "History and Introduction of Herbalism," a narrative that dives deep into the rich roots and expansive growth of this enduring tradition.

Spanning diverse civilizations, herbalism's story intertwines with ancient powers like Egypt and Mesopotamia, and stretches to the vibrant cultures of China, India, and further. This volume promises a deep dive into the annals of plant-based healing, urging you to traverse its illustrious timeline.

Within these pages, journey from the earliest inklings of civilization, witnessing the reverence with which ancient healers and sages tapped into nature, deciphering the potent curative abilities of myriad plants. Through exhaustive research and compelling narratives, this book presents a panoramic view of our age-old relationship with botanical remedies.

However, this isn't just a chronicle of the past; it's also a bridge to contemporary understandings of herbalism. In today's world, as we see a resurgence of interest in holistic treatments, there is a symbiosis of age-old traditions with modern-day science. "History and Introduction of Herbalism" positions itself as a guide, connecting the ancient wisdom with today's applications, enabling you to grasp and apply the transformative essence of herbs in today's context.

Venture deeper, and you'll meet plants that have left indelible marks on our shared history, from the calming chamomile to the venerable ginkgo tree. Master the ancient artistry behind concocting tinctures, brews, ointments, and more, harnessing their power to soothe, revitalize, and heal.

Whether you stand at the threshold of herbal exploration, are fueled by historical curiosity, or simply wish to foster a deeper bond with the natural world, "History and Introduction of Herbalism" awaits with a treasury of knowledge. Join us on this immersive odyssey, where the wisdom of yore meets the innovations of today, reacquainting us with the boundless healing potential of the verdant world around us.

# Chapter 1. Herbal Medicine in History

## The History of Medicinal Plants

For eons, mankind has turned to nature's bounty for curative solutions. From the insights of native tribes to the advanced healing methods of ancient realms like Egypt, Mesopotamia, China, and India, this section delves into the lasting influence of botanical medicine on human health and vitality.

- **Glimpsing Early Insights**: Dive into the understanding of primordial societies as they discerned the healing essence of flora and established detailed herbal healing modalities. Wander through the traditions of bygone herbalists and sages, whose legacies have woven the intricate fabric of botanical therapies.
- **Herbal Revival**: Observe the transfer of plant knowledge across societies, facilitated by evolving trade pathways and intercultural interactions. Track this herbal lore across regions, sparking a botanical revival that's etched in the annals of mankind.

## The Importance of Herbal Medicine

We plunge into the perpetual relevance of botanical cures and their pivotal role in holistic health. Highlighting its multifaceted benefits, we elucidate the continuous allure of herbal healing for those pursuing natural health avenues.

- **Wholesome Restoration**: Grasp the essence of herbalism, which perceives health as a symphony of body, mind, and soul. Recognize how this encompassing vision not only treats symptoms but targets the core imbalances affecting health.
- **Eco-Friendly and Organic**: Understand the environmental merits of using plants as medicine, underpinning sustainability and diminishing dependency on man-made drugs. Dive into the ethos of "eco-conscious healing" and the alignment of herbalism with eco-responsible values.
- **Empowering Self-Care**: Recognize the empowering nature of botanical medicine, enabling individuals to be active participants in their health journey. By harnessing knowledge and self-care rituals, one can foster a profound bond with nature, leading to conscious wellness decisions.

## Herbal Medicine in Modern Healthcare

Experience the blending of age-old plant wisdom with modern medical innovations, as herbal solutions complement established medical regimens, enriching healthcare.

• **Scientific Validation**: Engage with the escalating scientific evidence underscoring the potency of herbal cures. Acknowledge how detailed research and trials are spotlighting the medicinal prowess of flora, championing their acceptance in conventional medicine.

• **Collaborative Healthcare**: Learn about the merging of herbal expertise into standard medical realms, nurturing partnerships among herbalists, naturopaths, and medical experts. Appreciate the synergistic health approach that amalgamates diverse healing philosophies for enriched patient outcomes.

• **Individualized Attention**: Delve into the principles of herbal medicine that emphasize tailored, patient-focused care. Discover how herbal experts collaborate with individuals, weighing their distinct needs, habits, and inclinations to curate herbal regimens catering to their unique health demands. In our journey through the enthralling saga of botanical healing, we come to appreciate its timeless significance and evolving role in contemporary health spheres.

# Chapter 2. Herbal Tradition in the World

## Native American Medicine

Embark on a journey into the deep-rooted bond between indigenous cultures and the world of flora, where plants are not just medicines but revered spiritual companions.

- **Echoes of the Ancestors:** Dive into the legacy of Native American herbal practices, transmitted across ages. Understand their profound relationship with plant entities, the ritual of smudging, and the deep-seated respect for nature's therapeutic bounties.

- **Plants of Spiritual Significance:** Delve into key plants central to Native American healing practices, such as sage, cedar, tobacco, and sweetgrass. Grasp the significance of rituals, ceremonies, and sanctified processes that form the essence of indigenous herbal healing.

## European Herbal Medicine

Europe boasts an extensive lineage of herbal healing stretching across eras.

- **Herbs in the Medieval Times:** Travel to the era where cloistered gardens were the epicenters of botanical wisdom. Explore contributions from pioneering herbalists like Hildegard von Bingen and how monastic societies curated and employed botanical remedies.

- **Herbs of the Folk:** Step into the grassroots level of European herbalism, where common folk leaned on native flora and age-old customs for health solutions. Recognize the pivotal roles played by village curers, birth attendants, and green healers in nurturing and transmitting botanical wisdom.

## Ayurvedic Medicine

Dive into Ayurveda, a time-tested holistic health system birthed in the Indian subcontinent.

- **The Triad of Doshas:** Grasp the foundational idea of doshas – Vata, Pitta, and Kapha – and their influence on health. Delve into how Ayurveda employs herbs to rejuvenate and maintain equilibrium within this system.

- **Ayurveda's Green Treasures**: Get acquainted with the vast spectrum of botanicals and blends utilized in Ayurveda. From adaptogenic gems like Ashwagandha to digestive marvels like Triphala, immerse yourself in Ayurveda's rich herbal narrative.

## Chinese Herbal Medicine

Unravel the intricate tapestry of Chinese herbalism, grounded in millennia-old concepts of Yin and Yang, Qi, and the quintet of elements.

> • **The Herbal Compendium:** Dive into the expansive Chinese Materia Medica, a treasure trove of medicinal entities spanning plants, fauna, and minerals. Understand the essence of herbal synergy and the distinct diagnostic paradigms that define Chinese herbal practice.

• **Timeless Herbal Concoctions:** Familiarize yourself with enduring Chinese herbal mixtures, exemplified by classics like the Four Gentlemen Decoction and the Rehmannia Six Formula. Appreciate the art of formulating to address specific health imbalances, fostering holistic wellness.

## African Herbal Medicine

Journey into Africa's rich herbal milieu, where plants are both curative agents and revered spiritual guides.

> • **Rites and Remedies**: Discover the age-old healing modalities of African traditions, intricately weaving plant solutions with rituals, divinations, and sacred ceremonies. Understand the sanctity and therapeutic prowess of plants like Rooibos, Sutherlandia, and African Wormwood.

> • **Shamanic Heritage:** Grasp the central role of African shamans and traditional healers, custodians of deep botanical knowledge and applications. Explore the ceremonials, trance journeys, and communion with plant spirits integral to Africa's green medicine.

By journeying through diverse herbal legacies spanning continents, we deepen our appreciation for humanity's timeless liaison with curative plants. These global traditions underline the omnipresence of herbalism in healing physical, mental, and spiritual afflictions. The insights and rituals enshrined within these practices continue to enlighten and guide modern herbal enthusiasts, offering an integrative health approach deeply anchored in nature's bosom. As we navigate this mosaic of global herbal cultures, the confluence of ancestral wisdom and current insights beckons us, showcasing the immense prowess of botanicals in enhancing our health and spirit.

# Chapter 3: In-Depth Exploration of Herbal Systems

Herbal medicine has flourished in various corners of the globe, each having its distinct techniques, beliefs, and medicinal herbs. In this section, we'll delve into three prominent systems: Traditional Chinese Medicine, Ayurveda, and Native American Medicine. Each provides a unique perspective on healing, underlined by their practices and philosophies.

## Traditional Chinese Medicine: The Art of Balance

With millennia of practice, Traditional Chinese Medicine (TCM) offers a holistic approach focused on creating balance in the body, soul, and mind. Health in TCM is seen as a harmonious state, with illness being a result of energy disruptions. This system is grounded in:

- **Foundations of TCM**

Yin-Yang, Qi, and the Five Elements Drawing from nature, TCM uses the concepts of Yin (representing cool, feminine aspects) and Yang (capturing warm, masculine characteristics) as its foundation. The delicate balance between these forces is pivotal to health. Additionally, the flow of Qi or life force and the Five Elements theory also play key roles in understanding bodily functions and emotions.

- **Medicinal Herbs and Formulations in TCM**

The Chinese Materia Medica, a comprehensive herbal directory, is central to TCM. It introduces combinations of herbs that are meticulously chosen based on their qualities to rectify particular imbalances. Noteworthy herbs such as ginseng, goji berries, and ginger play pivotal roles in many formulations.

- **Integration of Acupuncture and Herbal Practices**

Acupuncture, another hallmark of TCM, is frequently used alongside herbal medicine. It involves the precise placement of needles to rejuvenate the body's energy pathways, enhancing the efficacy of herbal treatments

## Ayurveda: The Science of Life

With its roots in ancient India, Ayurveda focuses on the interplay between the body, mind, and spirit. This harmony is achieved through specific diets, herbs, yoga, and mindfulness practices. Key aspects include:

- **Doshas: Vata, Pitta, and Kapha**

Central to Ayurveda are the three doshas or energies: Vata (controlling movement), Pitta (overseeing metabolism), and Kapha (related to body structure). The balance of these energies is instrumental in one's health.

- **Panchakarma: Deep Cleansing and Renewal**

Panchakarma is a specialized purification method in Ayurveda. Through a sequence of treatments, it purges toxins, reinstates balance, and rejuvenates the body and mind.

- **Rasayana: Nourishment and Longevity**

Rasayana, the rejuvenation branch of Ayurveda, employs specific herbs and practices to nourish the body, boost immunity, and promote longevity. Herbs like ashwagandha and brahmi are staples in this practice.

## Native American Medicine: Healing Traditions and Plant Spirit Medicine

The diverse indigenous cultures of North America have a rich tapestry of medicinal traditions, which merge spiritual beliefs with healing practices:

- **Ceremonies and Healing Traditions**

  Spirituality is intertwined with health in Native American traditions. Ceremonies like drum circles, purification rites, and vision quests are conducted to realign individuals with the spiritual realm and foster healing.

- **Plant Medicines and Their Spirits**

  Plants, revered in these traditions, are both medicinal and spiritual. Sacred plants like sage, tobacco, and sweetgrass are pivotal for therapy. The spiritual essence of these plants is harnessed through rituals and prayers.

- **Land, Nature, and Preservation**

  Native American practices stress the intrinsic connection between human wellness and environmental health. They champion sustainability, ensuring both the health of nature and future generations. Their wisdom, transferred orally, strikes a balance between venerating old teachings and navigating present-day challenges.

# Chapter 4: The Role of Medicinal Plants in Contemporary Culture

In our modern, technology-driven society, many are rediscovering nature's healing capabilities. There's a growing trend towards using natural treatments, with an emphasis on botanical medicine, as a complementary health method. This section delves into the contemporary significance of medicinal flora in various facets of human life.

## Plant-Based Cosmetics: Nurturing the Skin Naturally

There's a rising demand for cosmetics derived from plants in recent times. People are becoming more aware of the ingredients they apply to their skin, and there's a movement away from synthetic options. Plant-based cosmetics present a wholesome alternative by utilizing the therapeutic qualities of herbs to benefit the skin. Ingredients such as plant extracts, essential oils, and infused herbs are chosen for their positive effects, and they're incorporated into numerous skincare items.

Such products hydrate, revitalize, and shield the skin without the addition of aggressive chemicals. Moreover, plant-based cosmetics champion environmental responsibility, as they commonly endorse organic cultivation and emphasize sourcing ethics.

## Herbs in Cuisine: A Mix of Taste and Wellness

Herbs have traditionally been employed to enrich the taste of food. But they're more than just flavor enhancers; they're also health boosters. Culinary herbalism focuses on integrating these plants into daily diets, aiming to delight the palate while also promoting good health. Different herbs come with their own health advantages, such as aiding digestion or reducing inflammation.

By adding various herbs to our food, we can benefit from their nutritional content and promote our body's self-healing abilities. Whether it's through fresh herb garnishes or herb-infused recipes, culinary herbalism introduces a dimension of health to our meals.

## Herbal Teas and Infusions: Sipping Nature's Remedies

The tradition of making and enjoying herbal teas spans many generations, serving both enjoyment and medicinal purposes. Herbal brews are produced by soaking parts of therapeutic plants, like leaves or blossoms, in boiling water. This method gently extracts the plants' beneficial elements into the drink, resulting in a tasty and health-boosting beverage. Herbal teas can offer a plethora of advantages, from relaxation to digestive support and antioxidant enrichment. With each herb offering its distinct attributes, one can customize their tea selection based on individual requirements.

## Herbal Nutritional Supplements: Filling Nutrient Shortfalls

In our current era, where processed diets and busy schedules might result in nutrient inadequacies, botanical supplements have become increasingly popular. They act as a solution, offering dense forms of medicinal herbs in formats like capsules or liquid extracts. These products provide a handy and potent method to bring the virtues of medicinal plants into daily life.

Different herbs cater to various health areas, from immune defense to stress relief and cognitive performance. When opting for botanical supplements, it's vital to ensure quality and adhere to the recommended intake.

## Herbal Medicine in Personal Care Products: Going Beyond Skincare

The value of medicinal plants isn't limited to skincare or culinary applications. There's a growing sector for personal care items that capitalize on herbal benefits. Ranging from hair care to oral hygiene and body treatments, botanical ingredients are diversifying their presence. Using these ingredients means opting for their healing, antimicrobial, and soothing properties, presenting a natural replacement for traditional products.

## Herbal Medicine and Mental Health: Nurturing the Mind

Mental health, an integral component of overall health, has always been aided by herbal medicine. This natural approach recognizes the profound link between the physical body and the mind. Certain botanicals, known as adaptogens, aid in managing stress, while others provide relief from anxiety or depressive symptoms.

Botanical solutions can also bolster cognitive capabilities, enhancing memory and concentration. Integrating botanical methods into mental health routines offers a natural and effective avenue for psychological support.

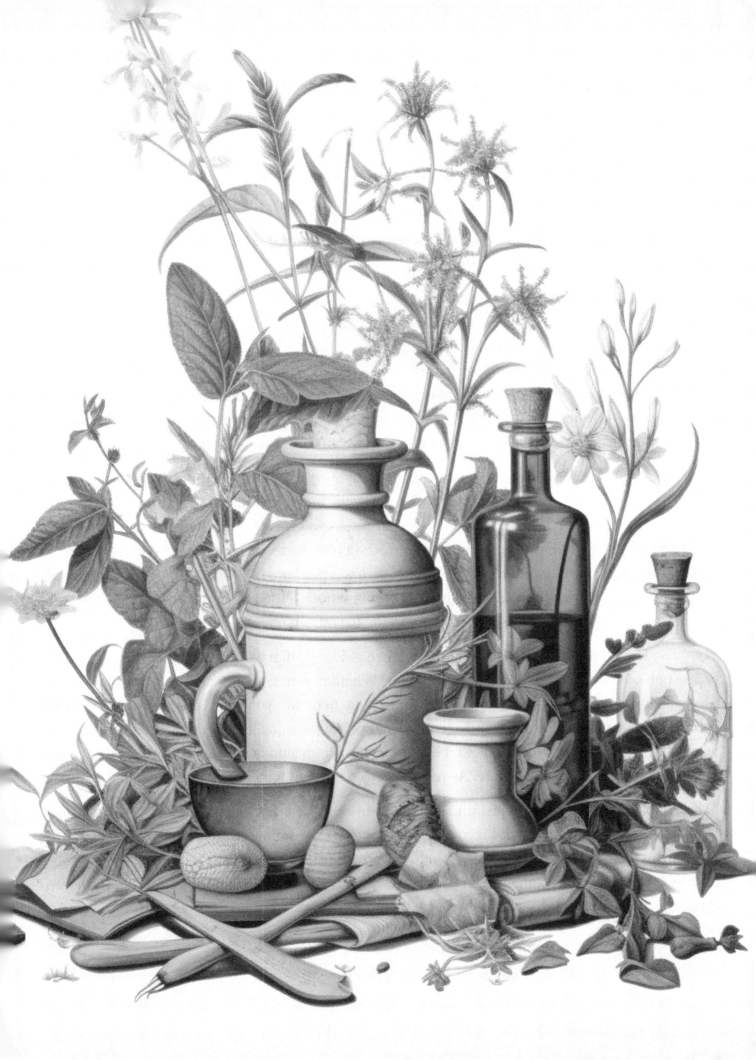

# BOOK 2: HERBAL APOTHECARY

## Introduction

Welcome to the enchanting realm of "The Herbal Apothecary," a guide that transports you through the wonders of herbal remedies and nature's wonders. In the subsequent chapters, you'll delve into the techniques and understanding of leveraging medicinal plants for holistic rejuvenation of body, mind, and soul.

"The Herbal Apothecary" stands as a bridge between age-old wisdom handed down across generations and the modern revival of herbology, captivating both the health-savvy and those drawn to nature's embrace. This extensive guide furnishes you with insights, curatives, and priceless suggestions to set up your very own botanical haven and set forth on a transformative path of self-nurturing. In our quest for true health, there's a deep-rooted desire for genuine, comprehensive solutions that sync with Earth's rhythms and recognize our intertwined nature.

The Herbal Apothecary addresses this longing by presenting a trove of insights on the planet's most potent and healing plants, enabling you to develop your individual herb collection and infuse the therapeutic qualities of these plants into your routine. As you traverse this book, you'll uncover the vast curative capacities of various plants, from the everyday herbs gracing our kitchens to the more elusive botanical treasures. Herein, you'll come across a plethora of herbal concoctions, spanning teas, elixirs, balms, and syrups. Through adept combinations of these herbs, you'll master the craft of herbal mixing, formulating potent blends specific to your unique requirements.

Yet, "The Herbal Apothecary" isn't just a reference guide; it offers you a pass to a transformative expedition of self-realization and empowerment. Whether you're a seasoned herb enthusiast or a newcomer to botanical medicine, there's something here for you. Its content overflows with actionable tips, inspiring stories, and age-old insights from various medicinal practices around the world, encompassing traditional Chinese practices, indigenous healing, age-old Ayurvedic knowledge, and European herb lore. As you set forth on this enlightening path, remember that

"The Herbal Apothecary" isn't just an assortment of remedies. It's a call to rekindle the timeless bond between us and the plant kingdom. It prompts you to immerse in nature's calm, heed the murmurings of the plants, and unveil the endless possibilities your personal botanical space offers. So, let the might of botanicals steer you towards robust health, profound ties, and deep metamorphosis. Approach "The Herbal Apothecary" with an open spirit and curiosity. Let your odyssey commence.

# Chapter 1: The Herbal Traditions around the World

## Traditional vs. Western Medicine

In the present day, Native Americans spanning various tribes frequently face a choice: adhere to age-old indigenous healing rituals or opt for contemporary Western medical therapies. Until not long ago, these two therapeutic approaches coexisted independently with minimal overlap. But today, Native Americans have comprehensive healthcare options at their disposal. Numerous traditional healers remain active within their tribal realms, and an increasing number collaborate with Western-educated physicians to craft tailored treatments for Native American recipients. Certain healthcare establishments even provide a blend of traditional and Western medical services. A segment of Native American individuals prefer receiving conventional healthcare from community-based practitioners rather than tribal health hubs. For instance, within the Mandan, Hidatsa, and Arikara (MHA) Upper Plains Tribes, members directly engage with local healing experts to avail their services. It's becoming common for Western medical specialists to recommend patients to traditional practitioners, and in specific scenarios, even aid in amalgamating Western and native healing techniques.

The cost of prescription medications has skyrocketed, rendering many out of bounds for a significant number who find them unaffordable. Conversely, herbal solutions, readily available in supermarkets and herbal outlets, are more pocket-friendly and typically have fewer side effects compared to pharmaceuticals. Even though the efficacy of many native treatments hasn't undergone rigorous scrutiny akin to pharmaceutical counterparts, they have proven beneficial in managing a spectrum of health challenges, from intricate conditions like arthritis and cancer to everyday issues like colds, coughs, and fevers. Historically, Native Americans resorted to chewing specific plant roots for ailments like colds, coughs, and headaches, whereas herbal teas addressed digestive discomforts. These botanical solutions remain accessible and can be home-prepared for a host of health concerns.

Numerous over-the-counter (OTC) drugs and prescription medicines owe their origins to components extracted from herbs integral to Native American healing practices. Thus, a substantial convergence exists between both the healing paradigms. Indigenous cultures have incorporated herbs in their diets, teas, and topical applications sourced from an array of plant parts like leaves, roots, and flowers. In contrast, Western medicine leans towards validated, industrially-produced pharmaceuticals.

Interestingly, several constituents present in today's medicines echo the ones employed by indigenous populations. This parallel isn't coincidental; modern medicine has extensively borrowed from, and remains indebted to, Native American botanical repositories. For instance, wild cherry, a prevalent constituent in contemporary cough remedies, has native roots. Native American communities have indubitably enriched global medical understanding. Numerous prevalent drugs, such as aspirin, quinine, and various cough syrups, incorporate nature-based elements, many pioneered by Native American traditions, that continue to revolutionize contemporary medicine.

## Native American Medicine

In our ever-evolving world, herbal medicine is experiencing a renaissance as a prominent alternative to conventional treatments. A myriad of practices, such as aromatherapy, acupuncture, and herbal therapies, stand as testaments to this resurgence. Herbal treatments, which utilize natural remedies, cater to a gamut of ailments and health concerns. These remedies can manifest as supplements, tea brews, essential oils, or powders. Clinical herbalists harness Native American herbs to tackle issues like arthritis, asthma, hormonal imbalances, and more. For these herbal solutions to be truly efficacious, they need to be accurately dosed, properly combined, and sourced from credible establishments.

While Western medicine, characterized by prescription drugs and surgical interventions, has made monumental strides in treating various ailments, it's not devoid of drawbacks. The side effects of some treatments can be debilitating, prompting individuals to seek solace in herbal alternatives. Aromatherapy, for instance, harnesses the power of scent to modulate one's mood, benefiting the mind, body, and spirit. The use of oils, flowers, and candles is prevalent in this practice. People's reactions to scents can vary dramatically. Consider lavender; its aroma not only soothes but also addresses respiratory ailments. On the other hand, basil invigorates the mind. Many fragrances rejuvenate the entire being.

Tragically, traditional or herbal medicines often languish in the shadows in numerous societies, primarily due to governmental and missionary-led vilification, sometimes even equating herbalism with witchcraft. Yet, despite such disparaging views, traditional medicines have displayed their prowess in remedying both psychological and chronic health issues, such as ulcers, bronchial disorders, and skin conditions.

Today, many modern practitioners are beneficiaries of the vast herbal knowledge bequeathed by Native Americans. Subsequent research corroborates that herbal treatments have the potential to address organic-based maladies. Emphasizing holistic healing, most herbal therapies encompass physical, emotional, and spiritual realms, underscoring prevention and inspiring healthier lifestyles.

Some argue that Native American movements have truly flourished by integrating modern methodologies and medicinal advancements. Traditional practices perpetually evolve, especially when applied within modern contexts. The stress-inducing urban lifestyle of today often sees solace in the arms of traditional healers, who bring to bear the herbal wisdom championed by Native Americans.

Herbalism offers remedies for a spectrum of conditions, from hypertension to dermatitis. As global appreciation for herbal treatments burgeons, many countries, from South America to Asia and

Africa, are endorsing a dualistic approach to healthcare. This paradigm allows individuals the autonomy to opt for herbal remedies or conventional treatments, or even a combination of both. A dedicated cadre of practitioners fervently champions herbalism, a tradition with deep roots in Native American culture. Those who experience the therapeutic virtues of these remedies often display a predilection for these natural solutions over synthetic ones, ensuring the continued relevance of herbal and Native American medicines in our modern age.

Herbal treatments can potentially diminish one's dependency on allopathic drugs, which often manifest as tablets or capsules. Unlike pharmaceuticals, herbs are not bound by stringent regulatory frameworks and don't necessitate exhaustive testing prior to market introduction. These remedies, being organic, are metabolized naturally, exerting gentle, predictable effects on our physiology.

All plants, by design, synthesize distinct chemical compounds during their metabolic activities. These compounds bifurcate into primary and secondary metabolites. While primary metabolites, such as fats and sugars, are ubiquitous across plants, secondary metabolites are confined to specific plant species or genera.

However, caution is paramount when venturing into herbal treatments. One must ascertain whether an herbal concoction will produce the intended effects without causing adversities. Individuals should ideally consult a physician for a comprehensive health check-up prior to commencing any herbal regimen. For instance, a hypertensive individual keen on integrating herbal remedies should be wary of potential interactions with prescribed medications, as they could precipitate drastic blood pressure fluctuations, with dire consequences.

In conclusion, the rich tapestry of herbal wisdom, with its origins in Native American traditions, offers a profound repository of healing. The intrinsic belief in the sanctity and therapeutic prowess of plants and herbs not only introduced the modern world to the potential of natural medicines but also underscored the spiritual symbiosis between humans and nature. Native American reverence for the healing attributes of plants serves as a beacon, illuminating paths to holistic well-being in our contemporary world.

## When to Use Native American Herbs

The nuanced world of Native American herbs, like any other therapeutic modality, hinges on individual variations and needs. Just as every individual reacts uniquely to medications, so too does their response to these traditional herbs differ. While discerning when to opt for herbal treatment over conventional medical care might seem intricate, there exist certain indicators that can guide one's decision.

Primarily, as a proactive measure, herbal medicine excels in fortifying the body at its foundational, cellular level. By fostering the creation of robust adaptogens, it enhances the body's innate ability to navigate and acclimate to environmental shifts and the vicissitudes of daily life.

In moments of medical urgency, prior to availing professional medical intervention, certain herbs can bolster the immune system. This heightened immune function not only underpins overall health but also equips individuals to lead fulfilling lives even in the face of daunting health challenges, including conditions as severe as multiple sclerosis, cancer, and AIDS.

One of the standout attributes of herbal medicine is its ability to amplify immune responses without causing unsettling shifts in an individual's state of well-being. This equilibrium cements its reputation as a stalwart methodology to nurture health holistically.

Nevertheless, like any powerful tool, herbal medicine can be a double-edged sword. Various reports have flagged concerns surrounding the health implications of certain herbs, with some even being relegated to "dangerous" categories. However, it's crucial to underscore that these apprehensions don't stem from the inherent nature of herbs but from their misuse. The pharmaceuticalization of herbs into pill forms often results in condensed, potent doses, which can be perilous if consumed indiscriminately. Like any therapeutic agent, herbs too have their threshold, and breaching it can precipitate adverse outcomes. Despite the infrequency of complications with herbal treatments, vigilance in adhering to recommended dosages remains paramount.

In summation, while the therapeutic allure of Native American herbs is undeniable, prudence in their application is essential. With mindful usage, these ancient remedies can serve as vital allies in our quest for holistic well-being.

# Chapter 2: How Medicinal Plants Work

Herbs boast distinct characteristics, enabling them to deliver a range of medicinal benefits. Each herb exhibits a mix of narrow and broad influences on particular bodily systems. Aligning an herb's traits with the health issues in question can holistically address the ailment, often leading to faster recovery with less consumption. By understanding these traits, one can interchange one herb with another.

Plant-based medicines originate from different sections of the plant like leaves, stems, bark, roots, flowers, and seeds. The therapeutic use of herbs remains widespread, with over one-third of Americans turning to them for various health concerns.

## Healing Properties of Herbs

Throughout history, cultures worldwide have harnessed the healing power of herbs. Ancient societies acknowledged the efficacy of remedies like white willow bark for fever alleviation, Echinacea for wound infections, and the toxic characteristics of hemlock and thorn apple. Such knowledge has been transmitted generationally through direct observation and experience.

Modern science now gives insights into the mechanisms by which certain herbs offer therapeutic benefits that were enigmatic to our forebears. This understanding is rooted in the identification of phytochemicals and enzymes in these herbs. These chemicals are products of the plant's metabolic activities.

Several phytochemicals, commonly used by Native Americans, act as robust antioxidants and bolster the immune system, effectively reducing cholesterol. Enzymes enhance these phytochemicals' effects, playing a pivotal role in the efficacy of herbal solutions. It's crucial to preserve these enzymes and not expose them to extreme heat or alcoholic solutions.

**Compounds in Plants and Their Benefits:**

- **Triterpenoids:** Found in licorice, they aid in liver purification and deter cavities and ulcers.
- **Diterpenes:** Romero is rich in these strong antioxidants.
- **Anthocyanidins:** Predominantly located in berries.
- **Salicin:** Sourced from white willow bark, used for flus, fevers, and persistent pains.
- **Lipoic Acid:** Detoxifies blood from heavy metals, shields the heart, and stabilizes blood sugar.
- **Omega-3 & Omega-6 Fatty Acids:** Essential dietary components that support the nervous system and reduce cholesterol.

- **Eleutherosides:** Enhance endurance and vigor, boost appetite, immune functions, and metabolic rates.

- **Flavoglycosides:** Antioxidants beneficial for blood pressure regulation.

- **Ginkgolic Acid:** Derived from Ginkgo Biloba, recognized for antioxidant, anticancer attributes, and aiding mood and mental sharpness.

- **Monoterpenes:** Powerful antioxidants from Ginkgo Biloba.

- **Hesperidin:** Common in thistle seeds; offers liver protection and fortifies blood vessels.

- **Saponins:** Anti-inflammatory, antibacterial, and antifungal agents prevalent in ginseng.

- **Isothiocyanates:** Powerful antioxidants located in horseradish.

- **Glycyrrhizin:** A compound in licorice known for its anti-inflammatory and antiviral effects.

- **Hypericin:** Helps stabilize moods.

- **Alkaloids:** Combat yeast growth, preventing infections and bloating.

- **Phenolic Acids:** Abundant in berries and flowers; they prevent nitrosamine production, a tumor-causing agent.

- **Phthalides:** Detoxifying agents in parsley with anticancer properties.

- **Chlorophyll:** Universal in green herbs, aiding wound recovery.

- **Gingerols:** Present in ginger, assisting in digestion and liver health.

- **Lactones:** Rich in kava-kava roots; they support cancer prevention through metabolic autophagy.

- **Elderberry:** Houses antioxidants known as proanthocyanidins. Renowned for flu resistance and cholesterol control.

- **Quercetin:** A metabolic enhancer noted in the "Sirtfood Diet" for its vast health properties.

- **Rosmarinic Acid:** Found in Romero; aids in alleviating nausea and migraines.

- **Silymarin:** An antioxidant in milk thistle, safeguarding the liver.

- **Tannins:** Plant compounds known for multiple health benefits, highlighted in the "Sirtfood Diet".

- **Polyacetylenes:** Parsley-derived compounds known for cancer prevention and regulating bodily processes.

# Chapter 3: Herbal Preparations and Applications

## Herbal Teas

Herbal teas present a delightful natural avenue to boost health and wellness. This section will delve into the health advantages of herbal teas and present various brewing techniques to harness the full therapeutic potential of these plants.

### The Benefits of Herbal Teas

Throughout history, herbs have been esteemed for their potential to enhance health and wellness. Every herb has its own set of attributes that cater to specific health needs. Here's a glimpse into a few renowned herbs and their health perks:

- **Chamomile:** Chamomile, with its tranquilizing attributes, is excellent for calming the mind, reducing stress, and encouraging restful sleep. It's a favored choice for those seeking relaxation, thanks to its gentle aroma and flavor.
- **Peppermint**: Bursting with freshness, peppermint assists in digestion, addressing ailments like gas and stomach discomfort. Its crisp menthol taste energizes the senses, making it a preferred post-meal beverage or a mid-day refresher.
- **Ginger:** Ginger, with its fiery undertone, boasts anti-inflammatory attributes and is sought after for its ability to counteract nausea and boost blood flow. Its warming nature makes ginger tea a comforting choice, especially on chilly days.
- **Echinacea:** Celebrated for bolstering the immune system, echinacea is a go-to for combating cold and flu symptoms. Its grounded flavor profile makes it a staple during times when one's immunity needs a boost.
- **Lavender:** Lavender's serene aroma aids in relaxation, improves sleep, and combats stress. Its subtly floral taste offers a calming effect, making it a nighttime favorite for many.

### Brewing Techniques for Herbal Teas

There are a few core techniques for brewing herbal teas, each designed to maximize the extraction of the plant's active ingredients. Here's a breakdown of the primary methods:

- **Infusion:** This popular method involves pouring hot water over herbs, allowing them to immerse for a set duration. This technique ensures the extraction of essential oils and other active components. The immersion time varies based on the herb and the intensity one desires. It's a straightforward method that promises a rich and aromatic drink.

- **Decoction:** Ideal for denser herbs like ginger or echinacea, this method necessitates boiling the herbs. The boiling process extracts the resilient components of tougher herbs, typically found in roots or barks. A lengthier brewing duration is needed to fully harness the plant's benefits, making it a method that truly taps into the herb's potency.
- **Cold Maceration:** This involves immersing the herbs in cold water for an extended period, often overnight. Especially apt for aromatic herbs such as lavender, this method retains their nuanced flavors and volatile ingredients. It's a patient process, perfect for those herbs whose active components might be compromised by heat, ensuring they retain their inherent goodness.

**Tailoring Your Herbal Tea Blends**

One of the delights of delving into herbal teas is the freedom to craft them according to your tastes. The versatility of herbs allows you to combine them in distinctive ways suited to your particular needs. For instance, a blend of chamomile and lavender yields a calming concoction, while ginger paired with peppermint results in an invigorating, digestive-friendly tea. You also have the leeway to determine the potency of your brew by adjusting the steeping duration; a brief immersion leads to a gentler taste, while a prolonged steeping intensifies the flavor.

To elevate the flavor, consider incorporating natural enhancers like honey or lemon. Honey offers a hint of sweetness and has its own therapeutic advantages, whereas lemon introduces a zesty note and aids digestion. Playing with various herb combinations and tweaking your brew gives you the privilege of designing a drink uniquely yours.

The realm of herbal teas is extensive and varied, brimming with a multitude of tastes, scents, and wellness advantages. Embrace the adventure of sampling new herbs, concocting diverse blends, and immersing yourself in the restorative essence of herbal teas. Relish the journey and cherish each flavorful gulp of your herb-infused creations!

## Tinctures

In this section, we'll venture into the intriguing realm of herbal tinctures. We aim to understand the crafting and application of tinctures, both internally and externally, and how they can be instrumental in promoting overall wellness.

## Crafting Herbal Tinctures

Tinctures stand as potent herbal elixirs, capturing the therapeutic essence of plants. They result from immersing herbs in solvents, usually alcohol, allowing the effective components of the herbs to be extracted. Their lasting potency and extended shelf-life make them highly esteemed.

## Preparing Tinctures

For crafting a tincture, you require herbs (either dried or fresh) and an apt solvent like vodka or grain alcohol. Here's your guide to the tincture-making journey:

1. **Herb Selection**: Aim for premium quality herbs that resonate with the health benefits you seek. Each herb presents unique properties; pick ones that cater to your requirements, such as ginger for digestion enhancement.

2. **Herb Treatment**: Clean fresh herbs, dry them, and then mince them to optimize extraction. If utilizing dried herbs, ensure they're uncontaminated.

3. **Ratio Calculation**: Set the proportion of herb to solvent. A popular proportion is 1:5, signifying one part herb for every five parts of solvent. However, this can be adjusted based on the herb and potency you're aiming for.

4. **Maceration Process**: Deposit the herbs in a glass container, drench them in solvent, ensuring they are thoroughly covered. Once the container is sealed and labeled, set it in a shadowy, chilled spot for a few weeks. Stir the mixture occasionally to foster comprehensive extraction.

5. **Extraction**: Post-maceration, sift the blend to isolate the herbal remnants, squeezing out as much extract as feasible. The liquid you obtain is your tincture.

6. **Bottling**: Pour the tincture into darkened glass containers, equipped with droppers to shield the concoction from light exposure. Label appropriately and stash in a cool, shaded spot. Handled this way, it remains potent for years.

## Employing Tinctures: Inside and Out

Tinctures offer a dynamic approach to tap into the curative prowess of herbs, with usage ranging from internal consumption to topical application:

- **Internal Usage**: For internal application, mix a minuscule quantity in water or a drink before consumption, ensuring quick absorption. Tinctures cater to diverse wellness needs, from aiding digestion to uplifting mood. Commence with minimal doses, augmenting as necessary, with the counsel of a trained herbal specialist.

- **Topical Application**: For external use, tinctures can be diluted with carrier oils like jojoba, crafting herbal-infused oils or applied directly. They can alleviate skin concerns, hasten healing, or address muscular discomfort. It's pivotal to execute a skin test before full-scale application.

## Safety Considerations

While tinctures generally align with safety norms, prudence is paramount. Some herbs might conflict with medicines or necessitate precautions under specific conditions like pregnancy. It's prudent to liaise with an informed herbal expert or medical practitioner to ensure tinctures are used safely and effectively.

## Salves and Balms

In this section, we'll journey into the domain of ointments and creams, understanding the process of designing therapeutic blends from medicinal plants for external use. We'll discuss the crafting, merits, and efficient application of these remedies for diverse skin concerns.

## The Power of Salves and Balms

Ointments and creams are topical concoctions blending medicinal plants with foundational ingredients like beeswax or base oils, yielding a product that rejuvenates and pampers the skin. Their role is to give specific relief, foster recuperation, and enhance skin vitality.

## Creating Healing Salves and Balms

Crafting personalized ointments and creams lets you shape the mixture to echo your desires. Here's a roadmap to this creation:

1. **Herb Choice**: Opt for herbs celebrated for their dermatological virtues. Calendula, chamomile, lavender, comfrey, and plantain are fine examples. Scrutinize the unique merits of each to pinpoint the optimal ones for your purpose.

2. **Base Creation**: Decide your mixture's base. Beeswax is favored for its consistency and moisturizing attributes. Base oils like olive or coconut play pivotal roles in infusing the herbs' benefits. Blend the melted beeswax and your selected oils over a double boiler.

3. **Herbal Infusion**: Integrate the herbs with the beeswax and oil blend, ensuring an even coating. Let it stew on a gentle flame, enabling the herbs to permeate the mixture. An alternative is to commence with pre-infused herbal oils.

4. **Filtration and Cooling**: After optimal infusion, sift the concoction, discarding plant remnants. After ensuring thorough extraction, let the resultant blend cool a bit, avoiding complete solidification.

5. **Incorporating Essential Oils (Optional)**: To amplify its aroma and healing profile, infuse essential oils. Opt for those that synergize with the herbs and bolster skin health, like lavender, tea tree, or frankincense.

6. **Filling and Solidifying**: Channel the lukewarm blend into sterile containers, like tins or glass jars. Let it set before sealing. Keep stored in cool, shaded spaces.

## Using Salves and Balms

These therapeutic concoctions cater to an array of skin issues:

1. **Skin Discomfort**: For minor irritations like rashes or sunburn, smear a delicate layer to quell and pacify.

2. **Minor Wounds**: After cleaning a wound, a dab can accelerate healing and guard against infections, leveraging the herbs' antimicrobial and restorative qualities.

3. **Moisturizing**: For parched or cracked skin, a little massaged in restores moisture and smoothness.

4. **Soreness Relief**: For aching muscles or joints, rub in gently. The herbs' pain-relieving and anti-inflammatory attributes offer solace. Always test a patch of skin first with a new product, discontinuing if reactions arise.

## Safety Considerations

Though generally safe, apply ointments and creams cautiously on open wounds or if you're allergic to any constituents. Always consult healthcare experts with doubts or known medical issues. By forging your own ointments and creams, you tap into the therapeutic prowess of plants, gifting your skin natural nourishment. Revel in this crafting journey and let these remedies be a tranquil haven in your skincare rituals.

# Syrups and Elixirs

This section will usher you into the enchanting realm of herbal syrups and elixirs. These rich, sweet blends offer both a delightful taste and a potent means to bolster immunity and overall health. Join us as we uncover the techniques behind crafting these natural tonics and the vast array of health advantages they offer.

**The Magic of Syrups and Elixirs**

Herbal syrups and elixirs are intense liquid solutions marrying the curative virtues of herbs with the sugary allure of natural sweetening agents. They're chiefly leveraged to fortify the immune system, mitigate coughs and aching throats, and as a comprehensive wellness enhancer. Their syrupy nature makes them especially inviting for those seeking a tastier health boost.

**Formulating Your Own Syrups and Elixirs**

Fashioning your personal herbal syrups and elixirs lets you fine-tune the taste and components, capitalizing on the therapeutic essence of herbs. Here's a sequential guide to crafting these tempting tonics:

1. **Herb Choice**: Settle on herbs renowned for their immunity-boosting or health-augmenting features. Favorites among many are echinacea, elderberry, ginger, and licorice root. Dive deeper into the unique attributes of each to align with your wellness objectives.

2. **Base Creation**: The foundational mix for these syrups and elixirs often involves water paired with a natural sweetener like honey or maple syrup. Gently warm this blend in a saucepan until the sweetener melds seamlessly into the water, tailoring the sweetness to your palate.

3. **Infusing with Herbs**: Upon preparing your base, introduce your chosen herbs. Allow this mixture to gently simmer for approximately 20-30 minutes, enabling the herbal attributes to suffuse the liquid. Periodic stirring will ward off any undue sticking or charring.

4. **Filtering and Cooling**: Post-infusion, set the mix aside to cool for a bit. Then, filter it to part ways with any herbal remnants, ensuring you extract all the infused goodness. Let your resultant syrup or elixir reach room temperature.

5. **Sealing and Storing**: Pour your cooled blend into pristine glass vessels. Mark them with details like the used herbs, sweetener, and date of creation. For maximum freshness and efficacy, refrigerate your concoctions, which, if stored correctly, can endure for weeks or even months.

**Using Syrups and Elixirs**

These herbal tonics can be wielded in several ways to amplify health:

1. **For Immunity**: In times of heightened susceptibility, like during flu seasons or exhaustion, a spoonful of these blends daily can serve as a shield, strengthening your body.

2. **Alleviating Coughs and Throat Ailments**: For these issues, a dosage can offer solace, dampening the irritation and pain.

3. **Everyday Health Boost**: Integrate these elixirs into daily beverages like teas, smoothies, or carbonated drinks for an added zest and health edge.

**Safety Considerations**

While these syrups and elixirs are predominantly safe, always be conscious of any specific allergies or intolerances to herbs or sweeteners. Before introducing them into your regimen, especially if you have ongoing health concerns or medications, seek guidance from a medical expert.

By mastering these syrups and elixirs, you open doors to a world where flavor meets wellness. Relish in the joy of making these enticing blends and let their restorative qualities uplift your health journey.

## Poultices and Compresses

In this section, we'll journey through the therapeutic world of herbal poultices and compresses. Renowned for addressing wounds, swelling, and muscle discomfort, these topical remedies lend direct relief while harmonizing with the body's innate healing rhythms. Join us as we unravel the art of their preparation and optimal application, showcasing their tranquilizing and restorative capabilities.

**The Healing Power of Poultices and Compresses**

Historically, poultices and compresses have marked their therapeutic stance in addressing various physical discomforts. They stand out by availing the direct touch of herbal mixtures on distressed areas, letting the skin absorb the curative wonders of herbs. While poultices are sculpted from damp components, compresses embrace hot or cold herbal brews.

## The Art of Crafting Herbal Poultices

Crafting an herbal poultice entails a blend of select healing herbs, typically dried and powdered, amalgamated with a binding damp agent. Here's a blueprint of the process:

1. **Herb Selection**: Opt for herbs renowned for their anti-inflammatory, anti-microbial, or calming attributes based on your specific ailment. Staples include chamomile, calendula, comfrey, and plantain. Delve into each herb's unique attributes to pinpoint the right fit.

2. **Herb Processing**: Transform the dried herbs into a fine powder using tools like a mortar, pestle, or a grinder. This helps unveil their potent essence, ensuring seamless skin penetration.

3. **Binding Medium**: To achieve the right poultice consistency, select a binder like water, herbal brews, aloe vera gel, etc. Mix this gradually into the herb powder until a dense, spreadable paste emerges.

4. **Application Method**: Directly layer the poultice onto the troubled region, ensuring a uniform layer spanning about ¼ to ½ inch. To bolster its efficacy, you can shield the poultice with a sterile cloth or bandage.

5. **Treatment Duration**: Keep the poultice affixed for roughly 20 to 30 minutes or as advised, allowing the skin to soak in the herbal wonders. Post-application, cautiously detach the poultice, discarding any residues.

## Creating Herbal Compresses

Herbal compresses hinge on the therapeutic touch of hot or cold herbal brews on the skin. They're versatile, apt for tasks like subduing swelling, easing muscle stress, or stimulating blood flow. Here's your guide:

1. **Herb Selection**: Your intended outcome will dictate the herb choice. Minty herbs like peppermint are ideal for a cooling touch, while fiery ones like ginger or cayenne suit a heating compress. Dive deep into each herb's profile for an informed choice.

2. **Brew Preparation**: For a warming compress, immerse the chosen herbs in hot water, steeping for 10-15 minutes. For a cooler variant, cold water suffices. Post-steeping, sieve out the herbs.

3. **Application Method**: Drench a sterile cloth in the brewed concoction, ensuring it's moist but not dripping. Press out excess liquid and place the compress onto the target area, adhering to your desired temperature.

4. **Treatment Duration**: Maintain the compress for around 10-20 minutes or as advised, letting the skin drink in the herbal essence. After the session, lift off the compress and dispose of the used infusion.

**Usage and Safety Considerations**

While poultices and compresses are typically benign, adherence to certain safety guidelines is pivotal:

• Prior to a full-scale application, a preliminary patch test can pre-empt potential allergic reactions.

• Refrain from applying on open wounds or cuts unless backed by a medical opinion.

• At any sign of worsening conditions or unexpected reactions, cease application.

• Especially for those pregnant, medicated, or with ongoing health conditions, a professional health consultation is advised before venturing into the world of poultices and compresses.

# Essential Oils for Aromatherapy and Topical Use

In this chapter, we'll journey into the captivating realm of essential oils, unearthing their process of derivation, their applications, and the holistic benefits they offer when used for aromatherapy and skin application. Derived from the heart of plants, essential oils stand as potent extracts cherished for their aromatic and healing prowess. Let's uncover the techniques of their extraction, delve into some notable essential oils, and embrace guidelines to wield them responsibly.

**The Art of Essential Oil Extraction**

Essential oils are nature's essence captured from different segments of a plant - be it the leaf, flower, stem, or root. The extraction methods vary, with the main techniques being steam distillation, cold pressing, and solvent extraction. Each process ensures the preservation of the fragile aromatic molecules that endow the oils with their characteristic aroma and therapeutic edge.

**Popular Essential Oils and Their Benefits**

1. **Lavender:** Revered for its tranquilizing aura, lavender essential oil is the quintessence of calm. It acts as an antidote to stress, offers solace to anxious minds, and serves as a lullaby for troubled sleepers.

2. **Peppermint:** A burst of rejuvenation, peppermint essential oil is the go-to for a mental reset. It eases throbbing headaches, sharpens cognitive faculties, and provides solace to unsettled stomachs.

3. **Tea Tree:** An ally for skin enthusiasts, tea tree essential oil stands as a powerful antimicrobial agent. It combats skin dilemmas like acne, fungal invasions, and minor abrasions.

4. **Eucalyptus:** Breathing made effortless, eucalyptus essential oil is a balm for congested chests. It declutters respiratory pathways, lends a fresh scent, and aids in unhindered breathing.

5. **Lemon:** A zestful delight, lemon essential oil radiates positivity. It's hailed for its purifying nature, mood-boosting capability, and its knack for instilling mental lucidity.

This list is just a sneak peek into the vast world of essential oils. Dive deeper to find the right aromatic companion for your unique needs.


## Safe Usage and Application of Essential Oils

When using essential oils, it is important to follow these guidelines to ensure safety and maximize their therapeutic effects:

1. **Dilution**: Given their concentrated nature, essential oils demand dilution. Employ carrier oils like jojoba, coconut, or almond as a medium for dilution when eyeing topical applications.

2. **Sensitivity Test:** Before a full-blown topical application, it's wise to initiate a patch test. Observe the skin's response to ensure compatibility.

3. **Aromatherapy Experience:** Relish the essence of oils via aromatherapy using diffusers or by infusing hot water with a few oil droplets. The aromatic journey promises relaxation, cognitive clarity, and mood elevation.

4. **Skin Application**: Post dilution in a carrier oil, you can apply essential oils to your skin. They find utility in skincare regimes, natural fragrances, massage blends, and aromatic baths.

5. **Storage Wisdom**: Guard the potency of essential oils by storing them in amber-colored glass containers in a cool, shadowed sanctuary.

## Safety Considerations

• Each individual's response to essential oils can vary. It's pivotal to recognize and respect any known allergies or skin sensitivities.

• Position essential oils beyond the reach of curious children and pets.

• Should you harbor health concerns, are on the path of maternity, nursing, or grappling with medical conditions, always seek advice from an aromatherapy expert or a trusted medical practitioner.

# Chapter 4: Creating Your Herbal Sanctuary

## Growing Medicinal Herbs

In this chapter, we shall unearth the magic and merit of nurturing medicinal herbs, be it in the tranquil ambiance of your garden or the cozy nook of your indoor space. Remember, a garden is an ever-welcoming confidante. So, brace yourself for an enlightening horticultural experience!

1. **Choosing the Ideal Herbs**: Prior to delving into the realm of herbal cultivation, it's imperative to handpick herbs that align with your unique requirements and the environment you provide. Some herbs bask in sunlight, while others bloom in dappled shade. As the age-old wisdom suggests, "Fit the plant to the place." So, evaluate the luminosity of your space and curate a list of herbs that resonate with those conditions.

2. **Laying a Robust Foundation**: Every gardener worth their salt will vouch for the vitality of fertile soil. To pave the way for your medicinal herbs to flourish, delve deep into the earth, smoothen the soil, and keep it free from detritus. Integrate organic resources like compost or aged manure to bolster the soil's texture and nutrient content. Bear in mind, "Nourish the earth, and in turn, it will nourish your flora."

3. **Mindful Planting**: Here comes the exhilarating phase - sowing your selected herbs. Craft planting pockets in alignment with the specific needs of each herb in terms of space. As you tenderly nestle the seedlings or seeds into their new home, visualize their journey to full bloom. The adage "From humble seeds arise majestic plants" reminds us of the potential latent in every tiny seed.

4. **Tending and Hydration**: Plants, akin to all living entities, thrive on care and compassion. Consistent hydration is paramount, particularly when Mother Nature turns the heat up. Heed the sage advice, "Quench the roots, spare the foliage." This ensures that water permeates to the core, rejuvenating the plant from its very base.

5. **Natural Defenses against Pests**: Every garden has its fair share of invaders. But, instead of resorting to chemicals, opt for Mother Nature's arsenal. Enlist the help of allies like ladybugs and lacewings that naturally prey on detrimental pests. Craft organic deterrents, be it a neem concoction or a potent garlic mixture, to keep adversaries at bay. Always remember, "Nature is the master cultivator," offering us green solutions at every step.

6. **The Power of Plant Companionship**: In the plant kingdom, companionship is akin to camaraderie—they mutually uplift and safeguard each other. Embrace the art of companion

planting to foster a balanced ecosystem. Interspersing aromatic herbs such as lavender or rosemary amidst other plants not only wards off pests but also infuses the air with their fragrant notes. The sentiment "Plants thrive in the company of friends" is epitomized in this mutualistic relationship.

7. **Reaping and Shaping:** As your herbs reach their zenith, the moment to glean their treasures draws near. Always pluck during the dawn, when the plant's essence is at its peak. Wield sharp tools to ensure neat trims, thus paving the way for robust regrowth. Regular pruning is a catalyst for lush, compact growth, preventing lanky stretches. Just as we evolve through life's trials, "Through trimming, plants burgeon with vigor."

## Harvesting and Drying Herbs

In this chapter, we will demystify the techniques of gathering and preserving herbs, ensuring that their healing attributes remain intact for your use. Echoing the sentiments of seasoned herbalists, "The essence lies in perfect timing."

1. **Picking at the Prime:** The secret to unlocking the medicinal marvels of herbs is to pluck them when they're brimming with potency. The perfect moment varies across herbs, often aligning with their flowering stage or when their aromatic oils peak. Embrace the adage, "In timing lies the magic." Picking too soon or too delayed can compromise the herb's taste and curative essence.

2. **Tender Gathering Methods:** Treat your herbal treasures with reverence to prevent harm or bruising. Utilize pristine, sharp instruments like shears or scissors, ensuring cuts are made just over a leaf junction or a lateral sprout. Evade rough handling that might drain nutrients or introduce impurities.

3. **Dawn's Embrace:** Mornings offer the golden hour for herb collection. With the sun's rays whisking away dewdrops and yet not strong enough to dissipate the essential oils, this time promises a rich harvest of aromatic and curative compounds.

4. **Preserving Plant Vitality:** As you gather, ensure the plant retains ample greenery to sustain its vigor and future growth. Abide by the guideline of sparing at least two-thirds of the plant during each harvest. This approach ensures the plant thrives through continued photosynthesis.

5. **Techniques of Preservation:** Drying is a revered method to safeguard the essence of herbs while prolonging their usability. Various drying techniques include:

- **Natural Airflow**: This technique requires forming herb bundles and suspending them inversely in a shaded, breezy spot. Ensure that the herbs are spaced out, preventing any fungal formation.

- **Dehydrator Use**: These devices offer a regimented ambiance for quick, yet gentle drying. Maintain a modest temperature setting (roughly 95°F or 35°C) to conserve the intrinsic qualities of the herbs.

- **Oven Technique**: In the absence of a dehydrator, an oven, set to its faintest warmth and left slightly open for airflow, can suffice. However, vigilance is crucial to prevent overheating, which can diminish the herb's virtues.

6. **Assessing Dryness:** The "snap test" is an effective gauge for dryness. Take a fragment of the dried herb and attempt to snap it. A clean break indicates optimal dryness, while any hint of moisture suggests further drying is needed.

7. **Storing with Care:** Post-drying, the sanctity of your herbs hinges on appropriate storage. Sealed containers, preferably of glass, shielded from direct light and varying temperatures, are ideal. Annotated labels with herb identification and collection date ensure you always have a reference for potency and freshness.

## Crafting Medicinal Herb Mixes

Crafting powerful herb combinations demands a deep grasp of each herb's healing traits and their synergies. Focus on the primary and secondary benefits of the herbs and their inherent qualities, such as warmth, coolness, dryness, or moisture. By merging herbs with harmonizing benefits and qualities, you sculpt a holistic and symbiotic blend.

**Choosing an Optimal Extraction Technique:** Different extraction techniques befit various herbs and expected results. Here are some prevalent methods:

1. **Infusions:** This technique involves submerging herbs in boiling water to draw out their healing elements. It's best suited for fragile plant sections like leaves and petals. As the adage goes, "Patience brews perfection." So, grant your infusion ample time to reach its full strength.

2. **Decoctions**: Best for the robust parts like roots, bark, or seeds. By letting these components simmer in water over an extended period, their therapeutic qualities are best harnessed. Embrace the wisdom of "Persistence yields results."

3. **Tinctures:** These are alcohol-infused extracts, giving a dense dose of herbal remedy. They excellently conserve and extract the herbs' active elements. Pick an apt alcoholic base, like vodka, and let the herbs steep for a few weeks. Indeed, "Great outcomes demand patience."

**The Craft of Herb Merging:** The objective when fusing herbs is to carve a well-balanced and synergistic concoction. Ponder the intended curative effect and the particular health issues you're targeting. Start with minimal herb portions, tweaking the ratios till you strike the right balance, abiding by the philosophy that "Perseverance refines skill."

**Balancing Flavor and Fragrance:** It's essential that herb combinations are not only potent but also inviting to the senses. Reflect on each herb's taste and smell. While some may lean towards bitter or sharp, others could be aromatic or sweet. Harmonizing these sensory aspects ensures a blend that's both potent and palatable.

**Maintaining Blend Records:** Chronicle the details of your herb combinations, noting the ingredients and their specific ratios. This not only aids in tracking efficiency but also refining formulas over time. With time, you'll curate a library of dependable recipes catering to various health needs.

**Customizing Blends for Individuals:** Recognizing the uniqueness of each individual, their health needs might demand distinct herb blends. Account for personal factors like age, overall health, and specific health issues when fine-tuning your concoctions. This bespoke approach amplifies the efficacy of herbal treatments.

**Diving into Age-old Herb Combinations:** Ancient herbal traditions, like Ayurveda and Traditional Chinese Medicine, boast their own revered herb combinations addressing diverse health challenges. Delving into these classic concoctions can illuminate enduring synergies and inspire your herb mix endeavors. As is often said, "In antiquity lies wisdom."

# Herbal Medicine Shelf

In this chapter, we'll delve into the crucial herbs and remedies pivotal for an all-encompassing herbal medicine shelf. Just as a kitchen thrives with a well-equipped pantry, natural healing pivots on a well-endowed medicine shelf. Let's unravel the hidden gems!

1.  **Cornerstone Herbs**: A select few herbs, given their diverse health perks, form the bedrock of any herbal medicine stash. Your selection should ideally encompass:

    *   **Echinacea**: A stalwart in bolstering immunity, especially handy during the cold spells.

    *   **Calendula**: Renowned for its reparative traits, it's an asset in ointments for skin woes and minor grazes.

    *   **Chamomile**: Celebrated for inducing relaxation, it's a remedy for sleep woes and tummy troubles.

    *   **Peppermint**: A cooling marvel, it assuages digestive glitches and curbs headaches.

    *   **Lemon Balm**: Its mood-enhancing and calming nature alleviates stress and fosters tranquility.

    *   **Ginger**: With its multifaceted benefits, it combats inflammation, nausea, and warms the physique.

2.  **Fundamental Remedies**: Along with the paramount herbs, your cabinet should be equipped with some foundational solutions. These can serve as independent treatments or be paired with herbs for diverse health needs:

    *   **Herbal Infusions**: Gentle teas crafted from dried herbs, ideal for relaxation or fortifying immunity.

    *   **Herbal Tinctures**: Potent extracts formed by soaking herbs in solvents, offering a convenient route to herbal healing.

    *   **Topical Herbal Preparations**: Balms and ointments that mend skin snags, minor burns, or insect nips.

    *   **Herbal Syrups**: Sweetened herbal concoctions, doubling as immune boosters and wellness tonics.

3.  **Emergency Staples**: Every herbal medicine shelf should be armed with basics to tackle standard injuries and afflictions:

    *   **Bandaging Essentials**: Imperative for shielding injuries and thwarting infections.

- **Natural Antiseptics**: Solutions like calendula or tea tree oil to sanitize wounds and expedite recovery.

- **Herbal Direct Applications**: Useful for immediate pain relief, inflammation curbing, and wound restoration.

- **Activated Charcoal**: A crucial remedy, especially for toxin absorption in cases of accidental poisoning.

4. **Reference Collection**: Housing a collection of trustworthy reference tools is equally vital. These can range from books to digital platforms, focusing on herb interactions, dosage protocols, and varied herbal cures for different ailments.

Building this collection is an evolving journey. By consistently broadening your knowledge and adapting your stash as per individual needs, you gear up to embrace natural, holistic well-being.

## Sustainable Practices

In this chapter, the spotlight is on the imperative nature of sustainable harvesting and the ethics governing medicinal plant use. As Earth's custodians, our duty is to uphold the integrity of these invaluable botanical wonders. Let's journey into the realm of eco-conscious herbalism.

1. **Mindful Harvesting**: The crux of sustainable harvesting lies in adopting measures that mitigate environmental impact and ensure the plant's longevity:

- **Plant Literacy**: Immerse yourself in the nuances of medicinal flora, from their growth patterns to habitats.

- **Conscious Gathering**: Harvest sparingly, ensuring the plant's survival and regeneration. Adhere to the principle: "Harvest with a gentle hand, leave ample for nature's plan."

- **Champion Regrowth**: Foster the cycle of life by facilitating plant regeneration and considering propagation methods.

2. **Nurturing and Preservation**: Home cultivation is an eco-friendly pivot from wild harvesting:

- **Opt for Locals**: Prioritize native or eco-friendly varieties suited to your locale.

- **Embrace Natural Farming**: Bid adieu to synthetic inputs, championing the health of both plants and planet.

- **Celebrate Diversity**: Diverse gardens bolster eco-balance and welcome beneficial fauna.

- **Seed Stewardship**: Uphold the legacy of plant diversity by mastering the art of seed conservation and sharing.

3. **Ethical Engagements**: Medicinal plant dealings come with an ethical compass:

    - **Cherish Indigenous Wisdom**: Revere the traditions and knowledge pools of local and indigenous communities.

    - **Combat Commercial Exploitation**: Strive for equilibrium between personal and commercial endeavors, ensuring eco-friendly sourcing and fair trade dynamics.

    - **Endorse Ethical Merchants**: Opt for suppliers championing transparency, sustainability, and just compensation.

    - **Circulate Knowledge Judiciously**: Share insights with humility, acknowledging origins, and fostering respect.

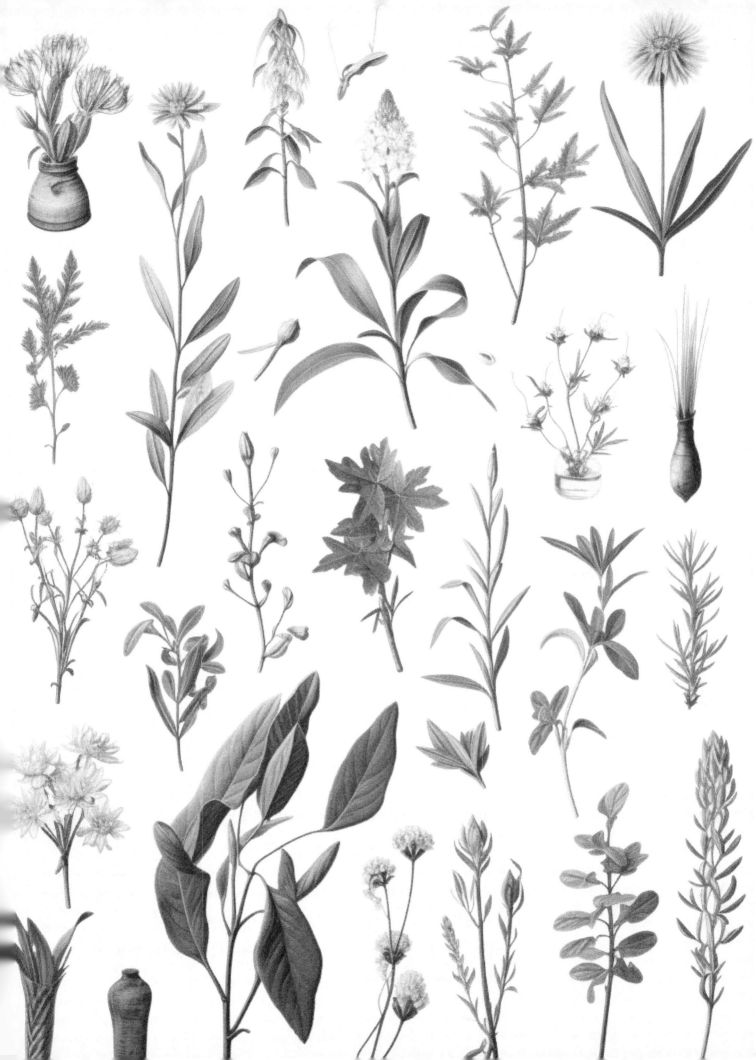

# BOOK 3: MEDICINAL PLANT

## Introduction

We invite you to step into the enchanting world of medicinal plants, a universe where nature's pharmacy reveals itself through vibrant hues, aromatic fragrances, and boundless therapeutic potential. This volume takes you on a captivating odyssey, immersing you in the vast world of botanicals and their significant contributions to human health and wellness. Within these pages, we discuss the remarkable capabilities of these plants, tracing their significance from ancient herbal practices to contemporary scientific insights.

From the earliest chronicles of human civilization, nature has been our go-to sanctuary for remedies, offering solace from ailments and a path to equilibrium. Different cultures, endowed with their distinctive practices and knowledge pools, have held medicinal flora in high esteem, integrating them seamlessly into their daily lives. This volume celebrates the time-honored wisdom handed down through ages, harmoniously merging it with contemporary medical advancements, bridging tradition with scientific inquiry.

Our expedition starts with a glimpse into the diverse spectrum of medicinal flora that graces our planet, from the verdant rainforests to the stark deserts. As we wander through nature, we unravel the secrets of various plant components, like roots, leaves, blooms, and seeds, and appreciate the unique healing attributes each brings to the table.

Subsequently, we immerse ourselves in the essence of herbalism, acquainting you with the core principles and hands-on techniques of employing plants for healing. To promote the sustained availability of these priceless botanical treasures, we underscore the importance of accurate plant recognition, ethical harvesting, and green production methods.

As we journey through this book, we shine a spotlight on the curative attributes of a myriad of plant species. Delving into their bioactive components, medicinal properties, and scientifically-backed applications, we introduce you to the healing wonders of both renowned plants like lavender and chamomile, and hidden jewels such as ashwagandha and ginkgo biloba.

Beyond their tangible benefits, these botanicals offer holistic nourishment, catering to our mental, emotional, and spiritual dimensions. Herein, we discuss how herbal remedies can be catalysts for relaxation, stress reduction, and emotional equilibrium. We stress the essence of fostering a deep bond with these plants and consciously recognizing their innate therapeutic essence.

This tome serves as a beacon guiding you through the intricate alleys of herbal healing. However, it's imperative to tread with caution and respect. Before embarking on any therapeutic regimen, especially if you're grappling with health conditions or are on medications, we fervently advise consulting a seasoned medical practitioner, herbal specialist, or naturopath.

This work aims to kindle your bond with Mother Nature and enhance your comprehension of the vast healing capacities of numerous plants. By valuing ancestral wisdom and juxtaposing it with modern scientific breakthroughs, we pave the way to harness the transformative might of our botanical companions.

Embark with us on this mesmerizing quest into the therapeutic domain of plants. Allow this volume to be your reliable guide, navigating you through the magical terrains of herbs, their curative prowess, and their overarching impact on holistic well-being. Our aspiration is to ignite your inquisitiveness, arm you with insight, and propel you towards the embrace of the botanical universe, catalyzing a healthier, harmonized existence.

# Chapter1: 55 Medicinal Plants

## 1. Arnica (Arnica montana)

**Healing Properties:**

Arnica stands out for its notable anti-inflammatory and pain-relieving attributes, making it a sought-after remedy for surface-level aches like bruises, twists, and muscular discomfort.

**Benefits:**

When used appropriately, Arnica offers multiple advantages such as alleviating pain, curbing inflammation, and aiding in the recovery of minor wounds.

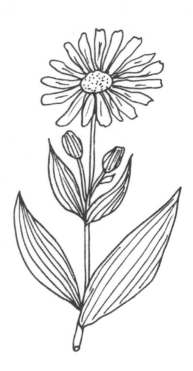

**Practical Applications:**

Arnica can be sourced in multiple preparations, be it gel, lotion, salve, or infused oil. It's pivotal to acknowledge that arnica is strictly for external application and should be put on unbroken skin only.

**Usage and History:**

Traditionally, Arnica holds a rich legacy in the annals of herbal treatments. Its legacy involves being topically applied to tap into its anti-inflammatory prowess, providing relief from pain and puffiness linked to bruises, strains, and muscular pains. It's reputed for potentially enhancing blood flow, thereby expediting the repair mechanism for wounds. On the other hand, internal consumption of arnica is generally advised against due to its harmful effects.

# 2. Ashwagandha (Withania somnifera)

**Healing Properties:**

Ashwagandha, an adaptogenic herb, is esteemed for its capabilities in alleviating stress and fostering holistic wellness.

**Benefits:**

Among the myriad benefits of Ashwagandha are bolstering the body's resilience against stress, amplifying mental acuity, rejuvenating energy, and instilling tranquility.

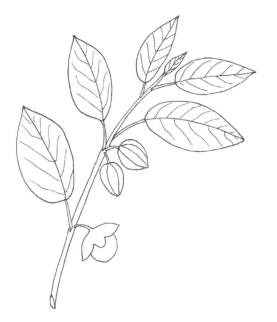

**Practical Applications:**

Most often, Ashwagandha is ingested in its powdered form or as capsules. Additionally, it can be infused as a tea or blended into beverages and health tonics.

**Usage and History:**

Central to Ayurvedic practices, Ashwagandha has been a cornerstone in Indian traditional medicine for ages. As an adaptogen, it plays a pivotal role in helping the body counteract stressors and maintain overall vitality. Over time, it has earned its reputation for reducing anxiety, enhancing cognition, energizing the body, and fortifying the immune system.

# 3. Astragalus (Astragalus membranaceus)

## Healing Properties:

Astragalus, a distinguished adaptogenic herb, is celebrated for its capabilities to fortify the immune system and bolster overall well-being.

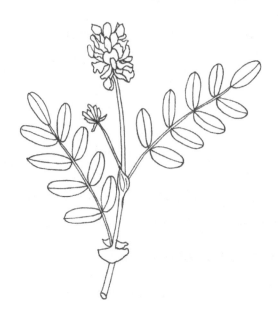

## Benefits:

The numerous benefits of Astragalus encompass immunity enhancement, revitalization of energy, bolstering heart health, and fostering a graceful aging process.

## Practical Applications:

Astragalus is versatile, taken as an infused tea, integrated into broths or dishes for its nutritional essence, or ingested as a capsule or tincture for ease.

## Usage and History:

With deep roots in traditional Chinese medicine, Astragalus is revered for its immune-strengthening attributes. Historically, it's been trusted to amplify the body's natural defenses and heighten resilience to various ailments. Often, Astragalus is paired with other medicinal herbs to boost vitality and optimize the health of respiratory, cardiac, and digestive systems.

# 4.Baikal Skullcap (Scutellaria baicalensis)

**Healing Properties:**

Originating from East Asia, Baikal Skullcap is an herb acclaimed for its antioxidant and anti-inflammatory characteristics.

**Benefits:**

Baikal Skullcap brings an array of benefits to the table: defense against oxidative damage, mitigation of inflammation, bolstering of liver functions, and fostering a tranquil state of mind.

**Practical Applications:**

This herb can be imbibed as a tea, ingested as a supplement in capsules or tincture format, or applied externally through creams and salves. Its antioxidant prowess and support for liver wellness make it a favored choice in many wellness routines.

**Usage and History:**

Rooted in the annals of traditional Chinese medicine, Baikal Skullcap boasts compounds with anti-inflammatory, antioxidant, and neuroprotective attributes. Historically, it's been sought after to treat a spectrum of ailments like respiratory issues, allergies, inflammation-related conditions, and liver-related disorders. Its tranquilizing essence is also noted, making it a remedy for anxiety and an aid in inducing relaxation.

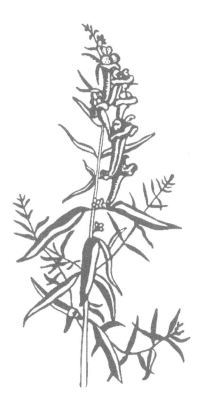

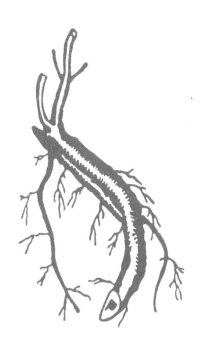

# 5. Baobab (Adansonia)

**Healing Properties:**

Baobab stands out as a superfruit, packed with an abundance of vitamin C, dietary fiber, and antioxidants. It's celebrated for its capacity to bolster the immune system and its anti-inflammatory characteristics.

**Benefits:**

The benefits of Baobab are manifold, encompassing bolstered immune responses, enhanced digestive function, revitalized skin health, and a natural surge in energy.

**Practical Applications:**

The powdered form of the Baobab fruit seamlessly blends into a variety of dishes— from smoothies and drinks to yogurts, even serving as a natural sweetening agent. For those seeking ease, it's also procurable in capsule format.

**Usage and History:**

The Baobab trees, indigenous to Africa, are revered not just for their fruit but also for their leaves and bark, all of which hold a place in traditional remedies. The fruit, brimming with vitamin C and antioxidants, is particularly esteemed for its immune-enhancing capabilities. Historically, Baobab has been a remedy for digestive woes, fevers, and infections caused by microbes. Not to mention, the tree's bark and leaves have occasionally been harnessed for their pain-relieving and anti-inflammatory potential.

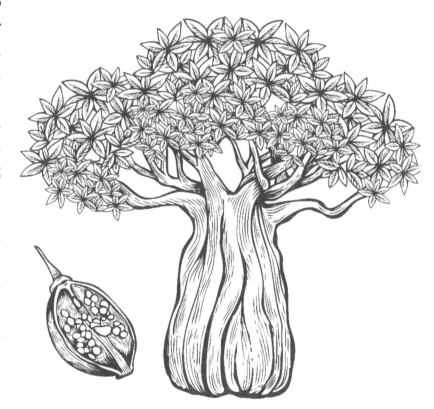

# 6.Black Cohosh (Actaea racemosa)

## Healing Properties:

Black cohosh is a therapeutic herb widely recognized for its efficacy in easing menopause-related symptoms, notably the occurrence of hot flashes and fluctuations in mood.

## Benefits:

The herb brings forth a plethora of benefits, encompassing hormonal balance, mitigation of hot flashes, enhancement of sleep patterns, and fostering emotional stability during the menopausal transition.

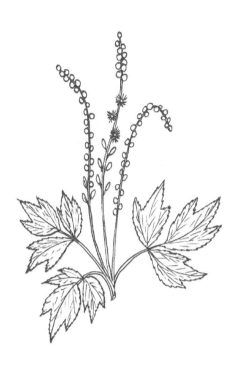

## Practical Applications:

Black cohosh can be sourced in diverse preparations like capsules, tablets, liquid extracts, and herbal teas. It's imperative to adhere to the stipulated dosage guidance.

## Usage and History:

Black cohosh has been anchored in the traditions of Native American as well as European herbal medicine for ages. Its predominant use has been to counter challenges faced by women during menopause, such as hot flashes, emotional roller-coasters, and disturbed sleep.

Attributed with properties akin to estrogen, black cohosh has been considered an alternative to conventional hormone replacement treatments. Furthermore, it's been tapped into for addressing menstrual discomfort and bolstering reproductive health in general.

# 7.Blue Vervain (Verbena hastata)

## Healing Properties:

Blue Vervain is a blossoming herb known for its tranquility-inducing and neural-supportive traits, making it invaluable for a range of ailments.

## Benefits:

Among its myriad benefits, Blue Vervain aids in curbing anxiety, fostering a sense of calm, alleviating tension-induced headaches, and enhancing digestive well-being.

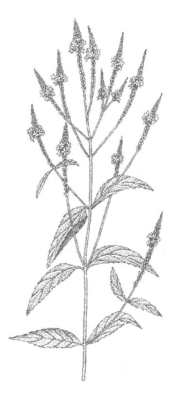

## Practical Applications:

The herb can be brewed as a tea, formulated into liquid extracts, or applied externally using a cloth soaked in its preparation.

It's predominantly sought after for its ability to soothe the nervous system and address digestive disturbances organically.

## Usage and History:

Embedded deep in the annals of Native American herbal practices, Blue Vervain is revered for its tranquilizing and sedating characteristics. This has made it a sought-after solution for dispelling nervous restlessness, anxiousness, and sleep disorders.

Moreover, with presumed pain-relieving and anti-inflammatory virtues, it has been tapped into for easing headaches and muscular discomfort.

# 8. Calendula (Calendula officinalis)

## Healing Properties:

Calendula stands out for its potent anti-inflammatory and skin-repairing attributes, making it a cornerstone for skincare.

## Benefits:

The plant offers a spectrum of benefits, encompassing alleviation of skin discomforts, facilitation of wound recovery, inflammation reduction, and potential mitigation of menstrual discomfort.

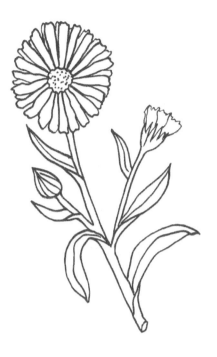

## Practical Applications:

Creams or oils imbued with calendula can be used on the skin to provide relief from an assortment of skin issues, such as minor abrasions, thermal injuries, and skin reactions.

In a different vein, a brew of calendula can function as a mouth rinse or gargle, catering to oral wellness.

## Usage and History:

Commonly known as marigold, calendula boasts a rich legacy in herbal medicine, owing largely to its unparalleled anti-inflammatory and skin rejuvenating attributes. Traditionally, it's been a go-to remedy for external skin afflictions like burns, wounds, and skin flare-ups.

Rooted in its capacity to aid tissue mending, diminish swelling, and soothe aggravated skin, calendula has garnered trust over time. Beyond this, when taken internally, it's attributed with potential germ-fighting and digestive-promoting properties.

# 9. California Poppy (Eschscholzia californica)

**Healing Properties:**

California poppy, a blossoming herb, is celebrated for its tranquilizing and analgesic attributes, making it ideal for relaxation and alleviating discomfort.

**Benefits:**

Incorporating California poppy into one's regimen can deliver diverse benefits such as fostering calmness, reducing symptoms of anxiety and sleeplessness, and offering gentle pain mitigation.

**Practical Applications:**

This plant can be enjoyed as a brewed drink, harnessed in a tincture, or ingested via capsules.

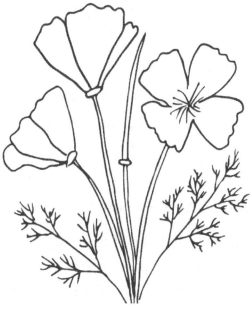

It is frequently sought after as a holistic solution for stress and disturbances in sleep.

**Usage and History:**

Indigenous to the Americas, the California poppy boasts a storied usage among Native Americans, primarily due to its calming and pain-reducing properties. Recognized for its ability to soothe, it has been an age-old remedy for conditions like anxiety, restlessness, and disrupted sleep.

Beyond this, it has also been a choice for mitigating various pain forms, including cranial and muscular discomforts.

# 10.  Cat's Claw (Uncaria tomentosa)

## Healing Properties:

Originating from the plant world, Cat's Claw is distinguished by its capabilities to adjust the immune response and counteract inflammation, making it an ally for bolstering the immune system and ensuring joint wellness.

## Benefits:

Among the myriad benefits of Cat's Claw are the amplification of immune responses, alleviation of inflammation, enhancement of joint ease, and fortification of digestive health.

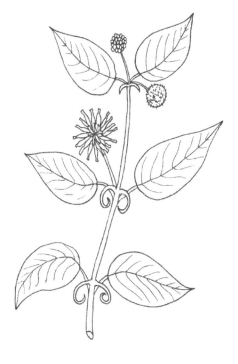

## Practical Applications:

Mostly found in forms like capsules, tablets, or tinctures, it's paramount to adhere to the suggested intake quantities and seek advice from a medical expert, especially when dealing with autoimmune issues or if one is on medications that suppress immune responses.

## Usage and History:

Hailing from the dense Amazon rainforest, Cat's Claw is a tenacious vine that's deeply rooted in the annals of traditional Peruvian practices. It's lauded for its knack to fine-tune the immune mechanism and combat inflammation.

Historically, it's been a go-to for enhancing immune robustness, mitigating arthritic discomfort, and tempering bodily inflammation. Moreover, its potential antioxidant properties are believed to enrich holistic health and vitality.

# 11.   Chamomile (Matricaria chamomilla)

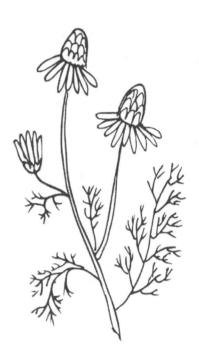

**Healing Properties:**

Famed for its tranquilizing and mollifying attributes, Chamomile serves as a natural panacea for stress alleviation and bolstering digestive wellness.

**Benefits:**

Chamomile boasts a plethora of benefits, such as mitigating anxiety, fostering a relaxed state of mind, enhancing sleep patterns, pacifying digestive upsets, and offering relief from menstrual discomfort.

**Practical Applications:**

A brew of Chamomile tea stands out as a preferred pick for those seeking serenity and restful sleep. This herbal infusion serves as a comforting drink.

Furthermore, Chamomile, when applied directly or infused in bathwater, can be a boon for various skin issues and expedite the wound healing process.

**Usage and History:**

Chamomile holds a venerable position in the annals of traditional practices from both Europe and Asia. Esteemed for its natural sedative and pacifying traits, it has been a household remedy for ages. Sipping on Chamomile tea is renowned for ushering in tranquility and fostering better sleep.

In the realm of external applications, it frequently graces skincare formulations, catering to inflamed skin and hastening the healing of injuries. Beyond this, its potency in assuaging digestive woes like gas and indigestion is noteworthy. This herb's holistic, gentle touch makes it an esteemed ally in nurturing comprehensive health.

# 12.   Damiana (Turnera diffusa)

**Healing Properties:**

Recognized for its sensual arousal and mood-elevating traits, Damiana is frequently sought after to amplify sexual desire and holistic vitality.

**Benefits:**

Damiana presents a spectrum of benefits, including fortifying sexual performance, enhancing emotional states, diminishing stress, and nurturing reproductive wellness.

**Practical Applications:**

This herb can be relished as a brewed drink or ingested as capsules or liquid extracts. Furthermore, it frequently graces various herbal concoctions and libido-enhancing mixtures, tailored to fit individual requirements.

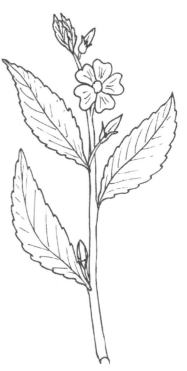

**Usage and History:**

Originating from the terrains of Central and South America, Damiana's roots trace back to the age-old practices of Mexican herbal medicine.

Attributed with sensual invigorating abilities, it's historically celebrated for augmenting sexual prowess and stimulating desire. Apart from its prominent role in sexual wellness, Damiana is lauded for its capabilities in elevating one's spirits, serving as a beacon of positivity.

Often steeped as an herbal infusion, its widespread inclusion in various herbal combinations underscores its esteemed position. On another note, this herb stands as a beacon of solace, offering relief from anxiety, despondency, and feelings of being overwhelmed, emphasizing its holistic benefits.

# 13. Dandelion (Taraxacum officinale)

**Healing Properties:**

Known for its detoxifying attributes, Dandelion's diuretic and liver-enhancing characteristics are instrumental for digestive vigor.

**Benefits:**

Dandelion's diverse benefits encompass fortifying liver functionality, detoxifying the body, aiding in digestion, reducing fluid build-up, and nurturing kidney vitality.

**Practical Applications:**

One can enjoy the freshness of dandelion leaves in salads or sauté them for an enriching meal.

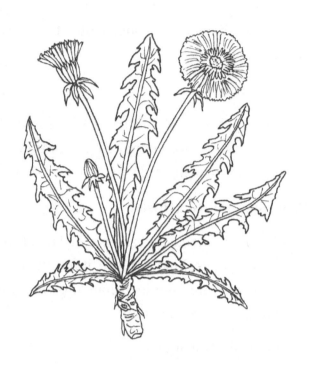

To derive benefits from its roots, people often prefer brewing them into a tea or opting for convenient forms like capsules or liquid extracts.

**Usage and History:**

With its deep roots in European and Native American healing practices, Dandelion is cherished for its ability to promote kidney and liver health.

By aiding toxin elimination, it plays a vital role in body detoxification. Its extensive mineral and vitamin content make it an invaluable health tonic, underscoring its prolonged and widespread use.

# 14. Echinacea (Echinacea purpurea)

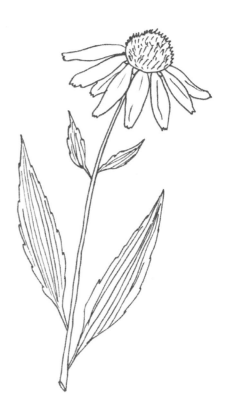

## Healing Properties:

Echinacea stands out for its capacity to fortify the immune system, hence it's commonly sought after for warding off and shortening the span of typical colds and respiratory ailments.

## Benefits:

The herb presents numerous advantages, encompassing bolstering immunity, lessening inflammation, and possibly assisting with wound recovery.

## Practical Applications:

One can drink Echinacea in the form of tea, opt for its tincture or capsule, or use it topically to benefit skin health.

This adaptability grants users the choice to assimilate echinacea in the manner they find most suitable and beneficial for their health regimen.

## Usage and History:

Originating in North America, Echinacea is a bloom cherished for its long-standing use, especially among Native American communities over the ages. Its esteemed reputation comes from its prowess in energizing the immune system, rendering a shield against ailments like the common cold, flu, and related respiratory issues.

It's speculated that Echinacea augments the efficiency of immune cells, fostering a sturdy immune defense. Accessible in diverse preparations such as teas, elixirs, and health supplements, it provides adaptability for users in choosing their mode of intake.

Its enduring application and acclaim underline its potency in buttressing immune wellness.

## 15. Elderberry (Sambucus nigra)

**Healing Properties:**

Elderberry stands out for its ability to fortify the immune system, making it a choice herb for potentially easing common cold and flu symptoms.

**Benefits:**

Elderberry boasts numerous perks such as curtailing the span and intensity of viral afflictions, bolstering the respiratory system, and delivering antioxidant defense to one's physique.

**Practical Applications:**

There are diverse modes to consume Elderberry, ranging from syrups, extracts to capsules. A crucial aspect to remember while picking elderberry commodities is to opt for those derived from heat-treated elderberries to circumvent any toxic effects.

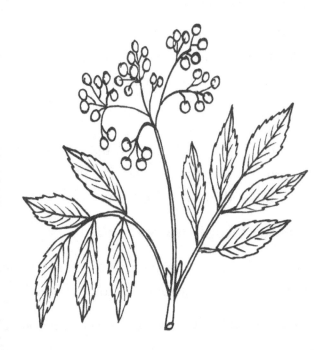

**Usage and History:**

With deep roots in classical European medicinal practices, Elderberry is celebrated for its berries loaded with antioxidants and capabilities to amplify the immune system.

Historically, it's been leveraged to diminish the length and acuteness of cold and flu manifestations. Its potential to thwart viral proliferation and kindle the body's immune response is noteworthy.

Popularly, people take elderberry in syrup form or infuse it in teas and concoctions, providing a spectrum of ways to weave this invaluable herb into one's health regimen.

# 16.  Elecampane (Inula helenium)

## Healing Properties:

Originating from Europe and Asia, Elecampane is a flowering herb known for its significant expectorant and antibacterial attributes, positioning it as an essential ally for respiratory well-being.

## Benefits:

This herb delivers a plethora of advantages. It aids in mitigating respiratory ailments, fortifies lung health, aids digestion, and enhances the immune system's defenses.

## Practical Applications:

There are myriad ways to harness the benefits of Elecampane. It can be steeped into a herbal tea, integrated into herbal concoctions like syrups or tinctures, or even inhaled through steaming.

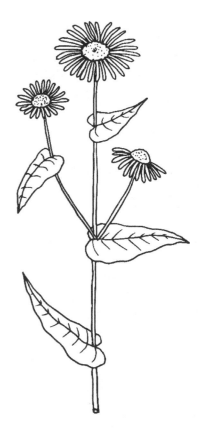

These methods are often chosen for bolstering respiratory wellness, particularly as natural treatments for conditions like coughs and bronchitis.

## Usage and History:

Throughout the annals of traditional medicine, Elecampane stands out, especially when addressing respiratory challenges.

Celebrated for its ability to ease symptoms such as coughs, bronchitis, and asthma, it's trusted for its mucus-clearing and airway-soothing attributes. Whether integrated into herbal mixtures or sipped as a tea, it's frequently chosen to enhance respiratory health and general vitality.

# 17. Eucalyptus (Eucalyptus globulus)

**Healing Properties:**

Native to the Australian terrains, the eucalyptus tree stands out with its distinct antimicrobial and expectorant traits, positioning it as a vital tool for respiratory well-being.

**Benefits:**

Eucalyptus offers a myriad of health benefits. It plays a role in quelling coughs, dissolving congestion, soothing sinus-related aches, and fortifying the respiratory system's overall efficiency.

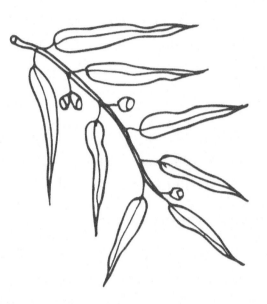

**Practical Applications:**

The essential oil derived from eucalyptus can be leveraged in diverse manners: from steam inhalation and ambient diffusion to being diluted with other oils for chest applications. One can also find its essence in common remedies like cough lozenges and topical treatments.

**Usage and History:**

With roots deeply embedded in Aboriginal medical practices from centuries past, eucalyptus has consistently been revered for its medicinal prowess, especially concerning respiratory ailments.

In contemporary times, the oil from the eucalyptus tree is either applied on the skin or inhaled to alleviate congestion, persistent coughs, and sinus-related challenges.

With its dual ability to clear breathing passages and fight respiratory infections, it's no wonder that eucalyptus oil is also chosen for topical use due to its pain-relieving and inflammation-reducing properties, granting solace from various ailments.

# 18.    Ginger (Zingiber officinale)

**Healing Properties:**

Famed for its potent anti-inflammatory and digestive qualities, ginger stands as a remedy for numerous ailments, notably in easing nausea and facilitating digestive processes.

**Benefits:**

Among its multifaceted benefits, ginger excels in mitigating nausea, diminishing muscle discomfort, and fostering a healthy digestive environment.

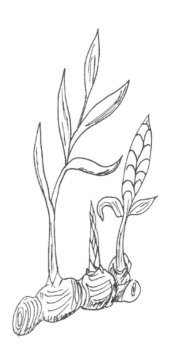

**Practical Applications:**

Ginger is versatile in its consumption, ranging from its raw root form to teas or even supplements. Beyond ingestion, it finds its way into culinary dishes or warm wraps to soothe muscle aches.

**Usage and History:**

Holding a revered place in traditional medicinal practices like Ayurveda and ancient Chinese remedies, ginger's legacy is underscored by its capacity to quell inflammation, promote digestion, and its characteristic warming nature.

Historically, it has been the go-to herb for issues like nausea, upset stomach, and other digestive woes. Furthermore, its anti-inflammatory traits serve as a balm for conditions ranging from menstrual discomfort to arthritis. Be it in its raw state, as a comforting beverage, or a culinary delight, ginger remains an enduring and cherished natural remedy.

## 19.   Ginkgo Biloba (Ginkgo biloba)

**Healing Properties:**

Ginkgo biloba, celebrated for its potent brain-boosting capabilities, is deeply respected for bolstering neurological health.

**Benefits:**

The tree offers a plethora of benefits, encompassing memory improvement, concentration enhancement, diminishing mental weariness, and fostering overall mental agility.

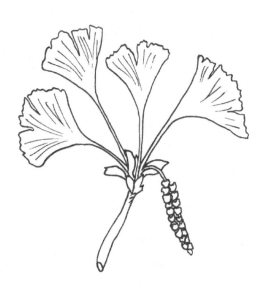

**Practical Applications:**

Most commonly, Ginkgo biloba is sourced in supplement form, often as capsules or tablets. Following prescribed dose guidelines, it's usually ingested orally.

**Usage and History:**

Ginkgo biloba, one of the most ancient tree species, occupies a revered spot in the annals of traditional Chinese medicine, boasting millennia of medicinal usage.

It's esteemed for its brain-strengthening virtues, including elevating memory, sharpening focus, and enriching cognitive prowess.

The tree is credited for promoting blood flow and guarding against oxidative stress. With a widespread presence in the supplement and extract market, its intake remains straightforward and accessible

# 20.   Gotu Kola (Centella asiatica)

## Healing Properties:

Gotu Kola, celebrated for its revitalizing and brain-boosting attributes, is esteemed for enhancing mental acuity and fortifying skin vitality.

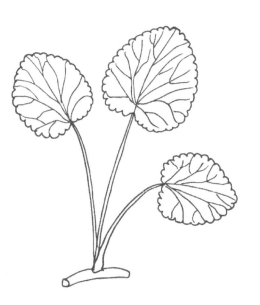

## Benefits:

Gotu Kola yields a multitude of benefits, encompassing memory augmentation, concentration enhancement, alleviation of anxiety, aiding in wound recovery, and fostering radiant skin.

## Practical Applications:

The herb can be ingested in diverse manners, be it through tea, capsules, or tinctures, granting multiple user-friendly intake options.

Furthermore, it serves a topical application, either as a cream or as an infused oil, beneficial for wound recuperation and treating skin ailments.

## Usage and History:

Gotu Kola is a distinguished herb in the realms of Ayurvedic and traditional Chinese healing systems. It has consistently been prized for its invigorating effects and its capacity to amplify cognitive performance.

Historically, Gotu Kola has been a go-to for bolstering cognitive abilities, refining memory, and achieving mental sharpness. Beyond the brain, it's recognized for its exceptional wound recovery qualities and its prowess in enhancing skin wellness.

Its consumption flexibility, from teas to topical ointments, underscores its versatile therapeutic reach.

# 21.  Hawthorn (Crataegus spp.)

**Healing Properties:**

Hawthorn, celebrated for its cardioprotective properties, stands out for its prowess in fortifying cardiovascular systems and augmenting blood flow.

**Benefits:**

Hawthorn boasts an array of benefits encompassing heart fortification, blood pressure modulation, circulation enhancement, and fostering a robust cardiovascular framework.

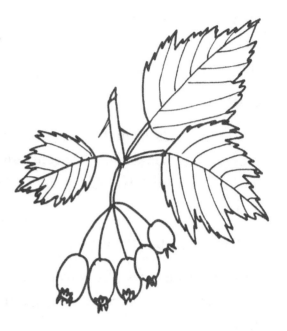

**Practical Applications:**

Hawthorn's berries, foliage, or blossoms can be utilized to craft teas, tinctures, or encapsulations, offering varied avenues of consumption. Regular intake is common as a preventive measure, cementing its role in sustaining heart vitality and overall circulatory health.

**Usage and History:**

Natively found across Europe, North America, and parts of Asia, Hawthorn, either as a bush or petite tree, carries significant weight in age-old European herbal traditions.

Its therapeutic use stretches back through the ages, predominantly in the realm of heart health. Treasured for their therapeutic benefits, Hawthorn's berries, leaves, and blooms have been pivotal in bolstering cardiac health, enhancing blood flow, and ensuring blood pressure remains in check.

The herb is attributed with properties like heart muscle fortification, cholesterol reduction, and bolstering general heart functions. Its wide availability, from infusions to supplements, empowers individuals to opt for their preferred intake method.

# 22.  Holy Basil (Ocimum sanctum)

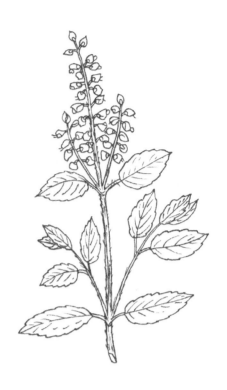

**Healing Properties:**

Also referred to as Tulsi, Holy Basil stands as a potent adaptogenic herb with an array of medicinal advantages.

**Benefits:**

Holy Basil, synonymous with Tulsi, brings forth numerous benefits encompassing alleviation of stress, bolstering mental acuity, immune system fortification, respiratory system sustenance, and digestive health enhancement.

**Practical Applications:**

Tulsi can be relished as a tea or ingested in encapsulated form, streamlining its integration into daily regimens. Its presence is also felt in culinary creations and various herbal concoctions, marking its diverse applicability.

**Usage and History:**

Venerated as a hallowed herb within the confines of Ayurveda, Holy Basil's therapeutic journey intertwines with traditional Indian medicinal practices, extending over millennia. Its esteemed adaptogenic traits and prowess in mitigating stress set it apart.

Holy Basil is celebrated for its capacity to sharpen mental focus, diminish symptoms of anxiety and depression, and uplift holistic health. Moreover, its curative scope spans respiratory ailment mitigation, immune defense amplification, and digestive system fortification.

Predominantly, Holy Basil finds its way into wellness regimens either as a soothing brew or in supplement guise.

# 23. Jiaogulan (Gynostemma pentaphyllum)

## Healing Properties:

Native to China, Jiaogulan is a twining vine renowned for its adaptogenic and antioxidant virtues, which amplify its medicinal significance.

## Benefits:

Jiaogulan encompasses numerous advantages such as mitigating stress, bolstering cardiovascular wellness, augmenting stamina, and strengthening the immune response.

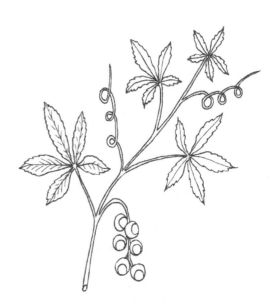

## Practical Applications:

Jiaogulan can either be sipped as a tea or ingested through capsules or tinctures, facilitating its seamless integration into daily habits.

Predominantly, it's harnessed as an adaptogen to elevate holistic health, amplify vitality, and bolster the immune system.

## Usage and History:

Often dubbed the "herb of immortality", Jiaogulan traces its roots to traditional Chinese therapeutic practices and is indigenous to China and parts of Asia. It's celebrated for its adaptogenic properties and its prowess in enhancing longevity.

Traditional beliefs credit Jiaogulan with optimizing cardiovascular wellness, modulating blood pressure levels, fortifying the immune defense, and aiding liver functionality.

Moreover, it's tapped into for its fatigue-fighting properties and its potential to enhance endurance. Be it as a calming tea or in the form of supplements, Jiaogulan provides myriad consumption possibilities.

# 24. Kava Kava (Piper methysticum)

## Healing Properties:

Kava Kava, native to the South Pacific, is acknowledged for its anxiolytic and calming attributes which enhance its medicinal significance.

## Benefits:

Kava Kava brings forth myriad benefits such as diminishing anxiety, fostering relaxation, mitigating stress-induced manifestations, and enhancing the quality of sleep.

## Practical Applications:

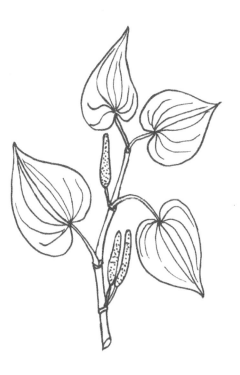

Commonly, Kava Kava is ingested as a drink formulated from its root.

However, it's imperative to approach Kava consumption judiciously, abiding by suggested guidelines, given its potential implications on liver health.

## Usage and History:

Kava Kava's usage is deeply embedded in the traditions of the Pacific Islanders, spanning over centuries. The plant's tranquillizing and stress-relieving virtues are widely acknowledged. Historically, it was leveraged to induce relaxation, ease anxiety, and instill a peaceful disposition.

Customarily, a beverage brewed from the plant's root was the chosen mode of consumption. However, it's paramount to employ discernment in Kava consumption due to its potential hepatotoxic effects.

# 25.  Kudzu (Pueraria lobata)

**Healing Properties:**

Kudzu, with roots traced back to East Asia, boasts therapeutic traits valuable for curbing alcohol cravings and alleviating withdrawal manifestations.

**Benefits:**

Kudzu proffers numerous benefits, encompassing the diminution of urges for alcohol, aiding detoxification, relief from hangover symptoms, and bolstering cardiovascular well-being.

**Practical Applications:**

Generally, the powdered Kudzu root or its extracts are ingested in the form of capsules or tinctures.

This is frequently woven into a holistic strategy aimed at alcohol addiction management.

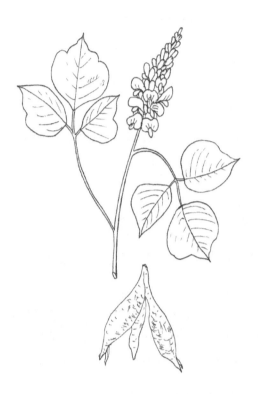

**Usage and History:**

Rooted in traditional Chinese medicinal practices, Kudzu has been revered for its curative virtues. The spotlight has been cast upon its potential in addressing alcohol-related cravings and the aftermath of overindulgence.

Kudzu root extracts are reputed to play a role in curbing alcohol consumption and assuaging the symptoms that emerge in the wake of alcohol withdrawal. Furthermore, its potential positive implications span areas such as heart health, symptoms of menopause, and digestive concerns.

Nonetheless, it's pivotal to recognize the need for more extensive research to decipher its true efficacy and ascertain its safety parameters.

# 26.  Lavender (Lavandula angustifolia)

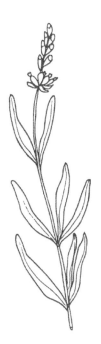

## Healing Properties:

Lavender, celebrated for its tranquillizing essence, is a beacon of relaxation and serenity. It's a frequent choice for mitigating feelings of stress and apprehension.

## Benefits:

The myriad benefits of lavender encompass enhanced sleep patterns, headache alleviation, relief for skin flare-ups, and soothing of minor aches.

## Practical Applications:

Lavender's essential oil, when dispersed in the surroundings, infused in bathwater, or applied to the skin (after dilution), champions relaxation and aromatherapeutic wellness.

It's also a delightful addition to herbal infusions and sachets, exuding a sense of calm.

## Usage and History:

Lavender's medicinal reverence spans centuries, boasting a legacy steeped in tradition.

It's lauded for its unique calming prowess. A staple in aromatherapeutic practices and herbal concoctions, lavender is instrumental in fostering relaxation, tempering stress, and fostering restorative sleep.

With its inherent sedative attributes, it is particularly adept at quelling anxiety, melancholy, and migraine episodes. Augmenting its portfolio is its antimicrobial facet, which, when used topically, offers respite from skin vexations.

# 27.  Lemon Balm (Melissa officinalis)

## Healing Properties:

Lemon balm, with its tranquilizing allure, stands as a testament to nature's ability to instill calmness and peace. It is a preferred choice for those seeking to mitigate anxiety and facilitate restorative sleep.

## Benefits:

From brightening moods to sharpening cognitive processes, from easing digestive grievances to assuaging symptoms linked with stress and unease, the plethora of benefits offered by lemon balm is vast.

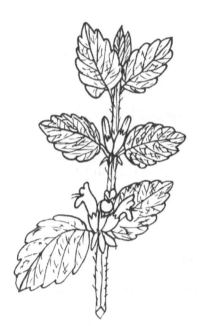

## Practical Applications:

For those seeking solace and restful sleep, lemon balm tea, crafted from either fresh or desiccated leaves, is a favored potion. Beyond its internal consumption, lemon balm can be administered externally as a soothing ointment or as an essential oil to calm skin agitations.

## Usage and History:

Rooted in European medicinal traditions, lemon balm has always been cherished for its capacity to calm nerves and elevate moods.

Traditionally, it's been an ally against anxiety, facilitating relaxation and endorsing deep sleep. Endowed with presumed antiviral and antioxidant virtues, lemon balm can be savored as an infusion or applied externally in an array of formulations.

## 28.  Lemon Verbena (Aloysia citrodora)

**Healing Properties:**

Lemon verbena, with its enticing citrus scent, boasts properties that soothe both the mind and the gut. Revered for its dual role in quelling anxiety and fostering digestion, it also stands as an ally in the quest for peaceful slumber.

**Benefits:**

This herb gracefully dances between various roles - from curtailing anxiety to fostering a relaxed state, from streamlining digestion to beckoning quality sleep. Lemon verbena is a multi-faceted gem in the world of herbs.

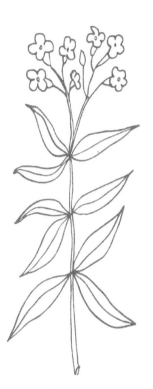

**Practical Applications:**

For those wishing to embrace the comforting embrace of lemon verbena, a tea made by steeping its leaves is the go-to choice. Beyond beverages, its aromatic presence makes it a delightful addition to various culinary creations.

Its versatility doesn't stop at ingestion; lemon verbena finds its way into herbal concoctions or is applied directly to the skin when transformed into infused oils, benefiting the skin's overall health.

**Usage and History:**

Having its roots in South America, lemon verbena has been an esteemed member of the traditional medicine repertoire, especially for its roles in aiding digestion and instilling tranquility.

Consumed chiefly as tea and celebrated in culinary realms, this herb has been trusted to ease digestive distress, such as bloating and indigestion, combat inflammation, and even ward off microbial invaders.

Beyond the digestive tract, lemon verbena has been sought after to ease anxious minds and ensure restful nights.

# 29. Maca (Lepidium meyenii)

## Healing Properties:

Maca, sometimes termed the "Peruvian ginseng", stands out as a potent adaptogen. Rooted deeply in the high plateaus of the Andes, it boasts an intrinsic strength that harmonizes hormonal ebbs and flows and fuels vitality.

## Benefits:

Maca wields a spectrum of benefits, ranging from invigorating one's libido to supporting reproductive health. Many hail it as a mood enhancer, a stamina builder, and a harbinger of hormonal harmony.

## Practical Applications:

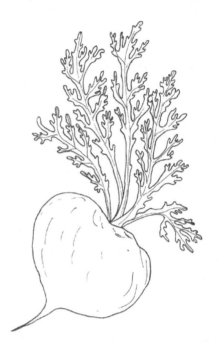

As a versatile herb, maca finds its place in our diets chiefly as a powder – a delightful addition to smoothies, a special ingredient in baked delicacies, or even a unique flavor in beverages.

Given its potent nature, it's prudent to embark on the maca journey with moderation, allowing one's system to adapt and determine the ideal intake.

## Usage and History:

Nestled in the high altitudes of the Andes, particularly in Peru, maca has carved a niche in traditional Peruvian healing practices. This potent adaptogen, with its multifaceted benefits, has been an ally in mitigating stress and fostering holistic health.

From amplifying energy levels to kindling passion, from ensuring hormonal equilibrium to easing menopausal and PMS discomforts, maca has been the go-to herb.

Today, this Andean gem is accessible worldwide, gracing health aisles in the form of powders, capsules, and other supplement variants.

# 30.   Marshmallow Root (Althaea officinalis)

**Healing Properties:**

Marshmallow root, a time-honored herb, stands out with its profound demulcent properties, providing a gentle balm for irritated tissues and mucous membranes.

**Benefits:**

Marshmallow root serves as a shield and soother for the body. It blankets mucous membranes, easing coughs and sore throats. Its prowess extends to bolstering digestive health, mitigating stomach ulcers, and fostering the healing of wounds.

**Practical Applications:**

Marshmallow root, in its versatility, can be harnessed in numerous ways. Whether steeped as a comforting tea, turned into a syrup for respiratory relief, or infused in topical concoctions like poultices or ointments, its therapeutic attributes shine.

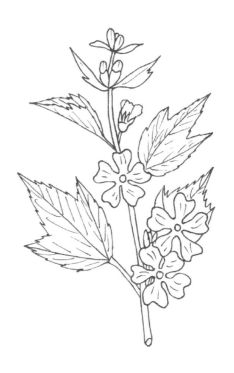

Predominantly, it's a stalwart in addressing respiratory woes, as it blankets and calms the mucous membranes. Beyond this, it emerges as a potent ally in gastrointestinal care, offering relief from discomfort and inflammation.

**Usage and History:**

Traversing back in time, marshmallow root's legacy is interwoven with traditional healing practices of Europe and the Middle East. Esteemed for its gentle yet effective demulcent characteristics, it has been the remedy of choice for a spectrum of ailments.

From assuaging sore throats and persistent coughs to mollifying respiratory irritations, marshmallow root has been the quintessential soother. Parallelly, it has been a guardian of digestive health, mitigating ulcers and other gastrointestinal disturbances.

In the tapestry of modern herbalism, marshmallow root retains its esteemed position, accessible in myriad forms, and continues to heal and comfort many.

# 31. Meadowsweet (Filipendula ulmaria)

## Healing Properties:

Meadowsweet, adorned with fragrant flowers, stands out for its innate analgesic and anti-inflammatory capabilities.

## Benefits:

Harnessing the power of nature, meadowsweet emerges as a relief provider for a variety of ailments. Its prowess includes alleviating pain, dampening inflammation, soothing digestive distress, and fostering a healthy urinary tract.

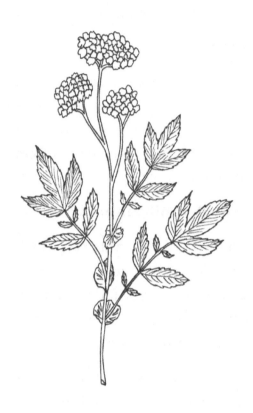

## Practical Applications:

Diverse in its application, meadowsweet can be crafted into a range of therapeutic products. As a tea, its aromatic essence provides both taste and remedy. Its efficacy also extends to its form as capsules, tinctures, or herbal extracts. Frequented for pain management, meadowsweet becomes a haven for those battling headaches, muscle soreness, or the aches of inflamed joints. Beyond this, its anti-inflammatory attributes offer respite for those grappling with inflammation. Moreover, meadowsweet, in its gentle approach, pacifies digestive disturbances and is believed to champion urinary tract health.

## Usage and History:

An herb of antiquity, meadowsweet's journey is deeply entrenched in European herbal traditions. Its salicylates, compounds mirroring the core ingredient of modern-day aspirin, render it its acclaimed analgesic and anti-inflammatory virtues.

Historically sought for its pain-dissipating abilities, meadowsweet was a remedy of choice for headaches, muscular tension, and inflamed joints. Furthermore, its potential in pacifying digestive woes and bolstering wellness has been well-chronicled. In contemporary times, meadowsweet's therapeutic tapestry continues to flourish, with its benefits being harnessed in myriad preparations and formulations.

# 32.   Milk Thistle (Silybum marianum)

## Healing Properties:

Celebrated for its distinctive liver-fortifying attributes, milk thistle emerges as a beacon of liver health support, safeguarding this vital organ from potential harm.

## Benefits:

Milk thistle's virtues span a broad spectrum. At its core, it stands as a guardian for the liver, defending against external toxins. Beyond protection, it fosters liver regeneration, mending and rejuvenating liver tissues. Its commitment to bolstering liver function is unequivocal, setting a foundation for overall health.

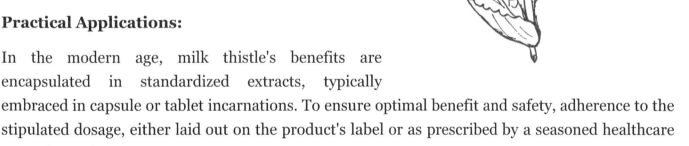

## Practical Applications:

In the modern age, milk thistle's benefits are encapsulated in standardized extracts, typically embraced in capsule or tablet incarnations. To ensure optimal benefit and safety, adherence to the stipulated dosage, either laid out on the product's label or as prescribed by a seasoned healthcare practitioner, is paramount.

## Usage and History:

Woven into the tapestry of European herbal traditions, milk thistle's narrative revolves predominantly around the liver's well-being. With a reputation as a hepatoprotective herb, it stands as a sentinel against potential toxins, shielding the liver from potential adversity.

The potency of milk thistle transcends protection—it is reputed for its capacity to facilitate liver tissue renewal, an essential aspect in maintaining liver vitality. Historically, this herb has been sought to ameliorate liver-centric conditions, such as hepatitis and cirrhosis.

In today's era, milk thistle's popularity persists, manifesting in diverse preparations like capsules, tablets, and infusions. It reigns as a sought-after herbal ally for liver fortification and detox. However, as with any botanical wonder, consultation with a healthcare maestro is advisable before embarking on its therapeutic journey.

## 33.   Moringa (Moringa oleifera)

### Healing Properties:

Moringa, often termed the "drumstick tree," is a veritable treasure trove of nutrients. Brimming with a plethora of vitamins, minerals, and potent antioxidants, it emerges as a formidable force for holistic wellness.

### Benefits:

Beyond mere nutrition, moringa's attributes are manifold. It invigorates, channeling a surge of energy to the body. It stands as a sentinel for the immune system, reinforcing its defenses. Digestion finds an ally in moringa, benefiting from its nurturing touch. The skin, too, rejoices in its radiance, fortified by moringa's nourishment. Moreover, its inherent anti-inflammatory prowess offers solace to inflamed tissues.

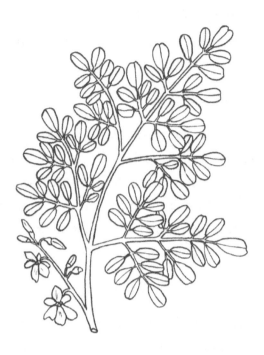

### Practical Applications:

Moringa's versatility shines in its myriad applications. The fresh green leaves can be incorporated into various culinary delights, from smoothies to salads. If fresh leaves elude, the dried or powdered form stands as a potent alternative, seamlessly blending into soups or juices. Those seeking a more concentrated dose can opt for moringa capsules, while teas offer a soothing alternative.

### Usage and History:

Rooted in the verdant landscapes of South Asia, the moringa tree is no stranger to traditional healing modalities. Ayurveda, an ancient Indian medical science, has long revered moringa for its therapeutic essence. Every part of the tree, be it leaves, seeds, or roots, finds a purpose, employed for its unique health virtues. Rich in essential nutrients, moringa leaves have historically been a source of vitality, enhancing energy and vigor. The immune system, too, finds solace in moringa's embrace, strengthened by its nurturing touch. Beyond immediate well-being, moringa showcases potential anti-inflammatory and antioxidant capabilities, proving its worth in mitigating inflammation and countering oxidative challenges. With heart health being paramount, moringa's influence extends to the cardiovascular realm, potentially offering protection and vitality.

# 34. Mucuna Pruriens (Velvet Bean)

## Healing Properties:

Often referred to as the velvet bean, Mucuna pruriens is a tropical plant renowned for its substantial levodopa levels, an essential component leading to dopamine production.

## Benefits:

This legume boasts a range of possible benefits like mood enhancement, cognitive boost, nervous system support, and fostering overall well-being.

## Practical Applications:

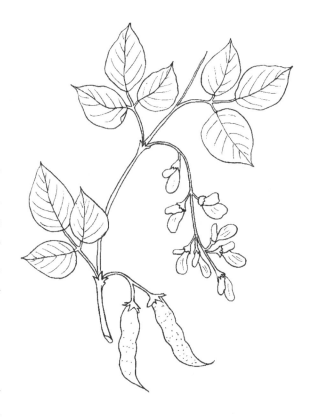

Mucuna pruriens can be integrated into daily routines in various forms. The powdered extract can be incorporated into drinks or meals. Those preferring a more regimented dose often opt for capsules or tinctures. When seeking natural means to enhance mood or cognitive performance, many gravitate towards this legume extract.

## Usage and History:

Traditionally rooted in Ayurvedic practices, Mucuna pruriens has been hailed for its positive impact on mental well-being. Its L-DOPA compound, a dopamine precursor, is instrumental in regulating mood. This has led to its study as a potential relief for Parkinson's symptoms, cognitive enhancement, and overall mood upliftment. However, its use requires prudence.

Before integrating it into a health routine, especially for those with existing health conditions or on medication, consultation with a healthcare expert is essential. Such professionals can offer advice on its suitable usage, dosage, and any probable side effects.

In summation, while Mucuna pruriens stands out for its prospective benefits in mental health, more in-depth studies are required to ascertain its comprehensive effects and functioning.

# 35. Mullein (Verbascum thapsus)

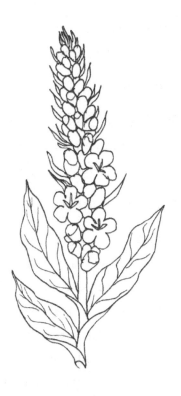

**Healing Properties:**

Recognized for its calming and mucus-clearing capabilities, Mullein plays a significant role in enhancing respiratory health.

**Benefits:**

Mullein is beneficial for easing respiratory problems like coughs, blocked airways, and discomfort. It also provides relief for a sore throat and aids in maintaining healthy respiratory systems.

**Practical Applications:**

To leverage its benefits, one can brew mullein leaves as tea, use them in steam inhalations, or convert into a tincture. It's a go-to remedy for breathing issues and as a natural mucus expeller.

**Usage and History:**

Originating as a flowering herb, Mullein has roots in both European traditional practices and Native American remedies.

Celebrated for its calming and mucus-clearing properties, it's been a trusted solution for respiratory issues such as coughs, bronchitis, and asthma. The plant aids in clearing phlegm and soothing inflammation in the airways.

A common preparation involves using mullein leaves for crafting teas or herbal concoctions that support lung health.

# 36. Neem (Azadirachta indica)

## Healing Properties:

Originating from India, Neem is celebrated for its capacity to combat microbes and calm the skin.

## Benefits:

Neem aids in maintaining skin health, treating skin problems like acne and eczema, expediting wound recovery, and enhancing the immune system.

## Practical Applications:

For practical applications, Neem is often incorporated into products like oils, creams, and powders.

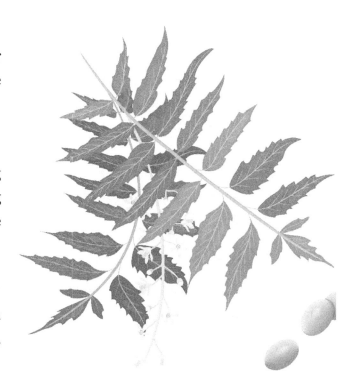

Its renowned antibacterial and antifungal attributes make it a favored choice.

## Usage and History:

Endemic to the Indian region, Neem boasts a rich legacy in Ayurvedic healing practices. It's esteemed for its multifaceted protective abilities, encompassing antimicrobial, antiviral, and antifungal actions.

Throughout history, Neem has been a remedy for diverse skin ailments, including acne, eczema, and various fungal issues. Beyond skin care, it is believed to bolster the immune system and has been tapped for oral and digestive wellness. Traditional cures often involve the use of Neem leaves, oil, or extracts.

# 37. Nettle (Urtica dioica)

**Healing Properties:**

Nettle, packed with vitamins, minerals, and antioxidants, is renowned for its therapeutic effects, especially in addressing allergies and joint concerns.

**Benefits:**

Nettle is believed to curb allergic responses, aid in managing inflammation, foster urinary health, and enhance joint ease.

**Practical Applications:**

One can drink nettle as a tea, cook it in dishes, or take it in the form of capsules or tinctures.

When handling nettle leaves, one should be wary of their stinging properties.

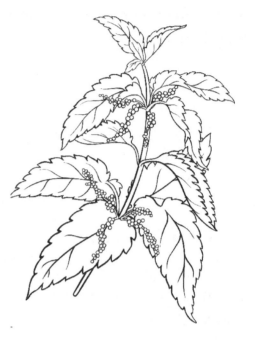

**Usage and History:**

Known to many as stinging nettle, this plant boasts an extensive past in folk medicine. Celebrated for its anti-inflammatory and diuretic characteristics, nettle has traditionally been employed to mitigate allergic symptoms, like hay fever, by decreasing histamine levels.

Additionally, it has found a place in promoting joint wellness, soothing arthritis discomfort, and enhancing skin health. Many prefer to consume nettle leaves in tea or use them in skin applications.

# 38.  Passionflower (Passiflora incarnata)

**Healing Properties:**

Passionflower is recognized for its tranquillizing and sedative effects, especially useful for those dealing with anxiety and disrupted sleep patterns.

**Benefits:**

It has the potential to lessen anxiety, induce relaxation, elevate sleep quality, and soothe nervous agitation.

**Practical Applications:**

You can enjoy passionflower as a tea, extract it as a tincture, or take it in pill form. It's crucial to stick to the advised dosage.

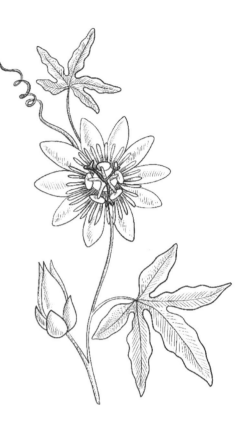

**Usage and History:**

Originating from the Americas, passionflower is a blossoming vine cherished in age-old remedies for its tranquillizing properties. It's typically sought after to counter anxiety, restlessness, and sleeping issues.

The flower is thought to boost GABA (gamma-aminobutyric acid) functions in our brain, aiding in relaxation and anxiety reduction. Its benefits can be availed through teas, tinctures, or dietary supplements.

# 39. Peppermint (Mentha x piperita)

**Healing Properties:**

Peppermint is recognized for its refreshing and calming qualities, often used to soothe digestive issues and mitigate headaches.

**Benefits:**

It assists with digestion, curbs bloating, alleviates tension-related headaches, and offers a revitalizing sensation.

**Practical Applications:**

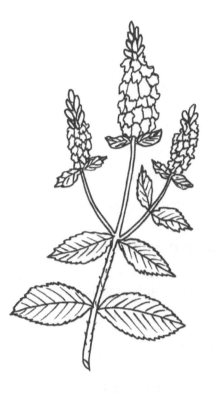

For benefits related to digestion, headache alleviation, and muscle relaxation, one can use peppermint in the form of tea, its essential oil, or as an infused oil.

**Usage and History:**

This hybrid mint plant, peppermint, holds a longstanding place in traditional remedies. Famed for its digestive and soothing properties, it's a common go-to for gastrointestinal relief.

Furthermore, its analgesic properties make it a popular choice for easing headaches and muscle discomfort. In modern practices, peppermint oil finds frequent use in aromatherapy and topical solutions.

# 40.   Prickly Pear Cactus (Opuntia ficus-indica)

**Healing Properties:**

This desert-dwelling plant, Prickly Pear Cactus, is celebrated for its anti-inflammatory capabilities and antioxidant-rich content.

**Benefits:**

The cactus might aid in maintaining blood sugar stability, fortifying the immune system, fostering good digestive health, and diminishing inflammation.

**Practical Applications:**

Both the fruit and pads of this cactus are edible and can be integrated into diets or formulated into supplements.

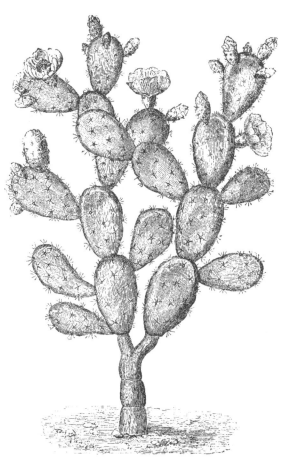

Its frequent usage centers around its rich antioxidant properties and its efficacy in resolving digestive disturbances.

**Usage and History:**

Historically rooted in Mexican traditional medicine, the prickly pear cactus is revered for a multitude of healthful contributions. Packed with essential vitamins, minerals, and dietary fiber, it's been a staple for regulating blood sugar, promoting heart health, and aiding digestion.

Both its fruit and pads are part of dietary practices, while its extracts find significance in age-old healing formulations.

# 41.   Red Clover (Trifolium pratense)

## Healing Properties:

Recognized for its abundant phytoestrogens, Red Clover is a blossoming plant with potential advantages in addressing symptoms of menopause.

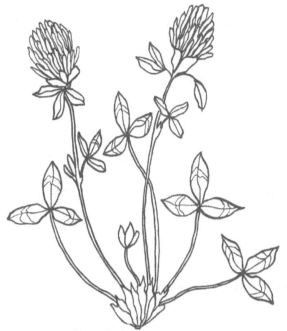

## Benefits:

Potential benefits include easing hot flashes, endorsing hormonal equilibrium, bolstering bone wellness, and fostering heart health.

## Practical Applications:

Regularly consumed either as a tea or in capsule and tincture variations, it's imperative to adhere to suggested doses and seek counsel from healthcare experts, particularly for those with conditions sensitive to estrogen.

## Usage and History:

Historically, Red clover has roots in both European and Native American medicinal practices. Esteemed for its phytoestrogen-rich content, it's been a go-to remedy for menopausal discomforts like night sweats and hot flashes.

Beyond that, its therapeutic properties have been explored for cardiovascular benefits and overall health enhancement.

# 42.   Reishi Mushroom (Ganoderma lucidum)

**Healing Properties:**

Reishi, an adaptogenic fungus, stands out for its abilities to both modulate immune responses and mitigate stress.

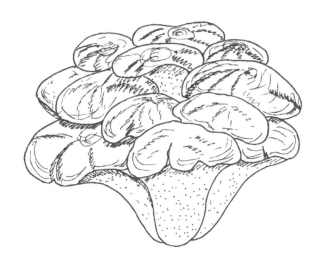

**Benefits:**

It's credited with bolstering the immune system, promoting better sleep, reducing inflammation, sharpening cognitive abilities, and fostering holistic well-being.

**Practical Applications:**

One can intake Reishi through teas, alcohol or hot water extractions, or in encapsulated form.

**Usage and History:**

Also referred to as Lingzhi, the Reishi mushroom is a stalwart in traditional Chinese medicine with a lineage spanning millennia. Celebrated as a robust adaptogen and an agent to modulate immunity, it's thought to augment the immune response, minimize inflammation, and invigorate the body.

Historically, its consumption is tied to aspirations of long life, better sleep quality, and cardiovascular fortitude. Its consumption varies from tea brews, powdered adaptations, to extracted formulations.

# 43.  Saffron (Crocus sativus)

**Healing Properties:**

Originating from the Crocus flower, saffron is celebrated for its potential to uplift mood and act as an antidepressant.

**Benefits:**

Saffron is believed to diminish depressive symptoms, uplift mood, sharpen cognitive faculties, and bolster eye health.

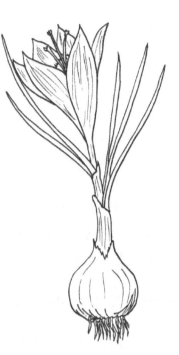

**Practical Applications:**

The vibrant saffron threads can be steeped in hot water or milk to craft a tea or be incorporated as a gourmet spice in culinary creations. Moreover, it's accessible in pill form.

**Usage and History:**

Sourced from the Crocus sativus flower, saffron has an extensive legacy in traditional healing practices. Recognized for its antioxidant and mood-elevating attributes, it has been historically prescribed to counteract depression, elevate spirits, and curb anxiety.

Furthermore, its purported benefits extend to eye health, brain functionality, and relief from menstrual discomforts. While used judiciously in cooking, saffron can also be ingested as a dietary supplement.

# 44.  Sage (Salvia officinalis)

**Healing Properties:**

Renowned for its antibacterial, antifungal, and anti-inflammatory characteristics, sage is a boon for oral hygiene and overall health.

**Benefits:**

Sage may provide relief for sore throats, ease symptoms of menopause, bolster memory and cognitive capacities, and foster digestive wellness.

**Practical Applications:**

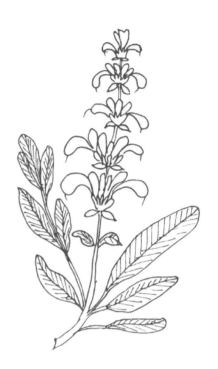

While sage is a popular culinary herb, it can also be steeped as tea or employed as a mouthwash to maintain oral hygiene. For those seeking alternative forms, sage is available in tinctures or pills..

**Usage and History:**

Esteemed for its medicinal virtues for many eras, sage has been a staple in both European and Native American traditional remedies. Celebrated for its antimicrobial and soothing abilities, it's been utilized to nurture oral health, soothe throat pain, and aid digestion.

Moreover, it's considered beneficial for the brain, enhancing memory and focus. Beyond its medicinal uses, sage leaves are versatile, finding their way into culinary dishes, teas, and various herbal concoctions.

# 45. Saw Palmetto (Serenoa repens)

## Healing Properties:

Saw palmetto is chiefly recognized for promoting prostate health among men.

## Benefits:

It can potentially alleviate signs of an enlarged prostate, including frequent urges to urinate and challenges in the urination process.

## Practical Applications:

Generally taken as a standardized extract, saw palmetto is available in capsule or tablet formats. Adhering to the suggested dose is crucial.

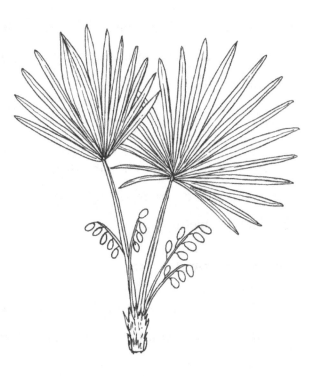

## Usage and History:

Originating from North America, saw palmetto is a diminutive palm tree with roots in Native American medicinal practices, specifically for prostate health support.

Frequently employed to lessen symptoms linked to benign prostatic hyperplasia (BPH) such as increased urination and urination challenges, it's theorized that saw palmetto obstructs the transformation of testosterone into dihydrotestosterone (DHT) while curbing prostate inflammation. Extracts of saw palmetto are popularly incorporated into supplements.

# 46.   Schisandra (Schisandra chinensis)

**Healing Properties:**

Schisandra is a renowned adaptogenic berry, celebrated for its capacity to invigorate vitality and bolster overall well-being.

**Benefits:**

Potential benefits encompass elevated energy levels, diminished fatigue, fortified liver functionality, enhanced cognitive prowess, and a general feeling of wellness.

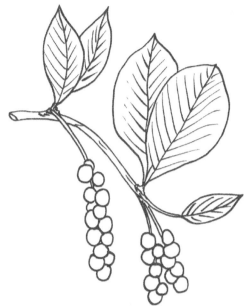

**Practical Applications:**

The berries of Schisandra can be brewed into a tea, hot water-extracted, or consumed in the form of a capsule or tincture.

**Usage and History:**

Originating in China, Schisandra is a vine that has been integral to traditional Chinese medicine across many generations.

As an adaptogen, it's championed for amplifying the body's innate ability to combat stress while fostering a sense of vitality. Traditionally, it's leveraged to bolster mental acuity, prolong stamina, nurture liver health, and counteract fatigue. Consumables like teas or extracts often incorporate Schisandra.

# 47. Skullcap (Scutellaria lateriflora)

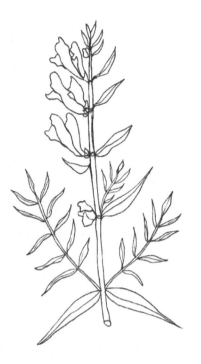

**Healing Properties:**

Skullcap stands out for its inherent calming and sedative properties.

**Benefits:**

This herb potentially aids in diminishing anxiety, fostering relaxation, mitigating nervous tension, and facilitating restful sleep.

**Practical Applications:**

Skullcap can be brewed into a tea, transformed into a tincture, or encapsulated. Owing to its natural sedative traits, it's frequently recommended for issues like anxiety and sleep disturbances.

**Usage and History:**

Hailing from North America, Skullcap has woven its way into traditional Native American as well as Western herbal medicinal practices. Valued for its soothing effects, it's been a go-to remedy for conditions like anxiety, unease, and sleeplessness.

Additionally, Skullcap is revered for its potential anti-inflammatory and antioxidant capacities. Whether brewed as a calming tea or consumed as a supplement, its benefits can be manifold.

# 48. Solomon's Seal (Polygonatum biflorum)

**Healing Properties:**

Solomon's Seal, a perennial herb originating from North America, is recognized for its potent anti-inflammatory and bone-mending properties.

**Benefits:**

This herb can potentially alleviate joint discomfort, bolster musculoskeletal health, aid in digestion, and enhance skin health.

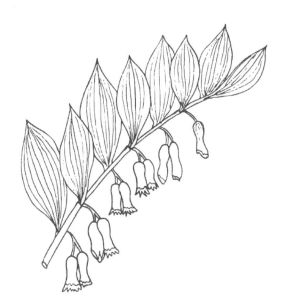

**Practical Applications:**

Solomon's Seal can be brewed into a revitalizing tea, processed into tinctures, or applied topically using poultices or salves. Given its inherent anti-inflammatory attributes, it is frequently advocated for joint and bone health.

**Usage and History:**

Deeply rooted in the annals of various medicinal traditions, Solomon's Seal has been a staple in practices like Traditional Chinese Medicine (TCM) and indigenous Native American remedies. Particularly revered for its potential to fortify joint and bone health, Solomon's Seal has historically been a remedy for joint aches, inflammation, and arthritic conditions.

Further, it finds mention for its potential digestive benefits, aiding respiratory function, and expediting the wound healing process. Various elements of the plant, particularly its roots and rhizomes, are prized for their medicinal value.

# 49.    St. John's Wort (Hypericum perforatum)

## Healing Properties:

Recognized for its mood-enhancing and potential antidepressant qualities, St. John's Wort has traditionally been a beacon for those seeking emotional balance.

## Benefits:

The herb is believed to be effective in alleviating symptoms associated with mild to moderate depression. It has the potential to uplift one's mood and foster emotional equilibrium.

## Practical Applications:

You can intake St. John's Wort in capsule form or as a tincture. Given the possibility of interactions with other medications, it's paramount to consult a healthcare practitioner prior to its use.

## Usage and History:

Originating as a flowering herb, St. John's Wort boasts a rich legacy in European traditional medicinal practices. Its repute primarily stems from its purported antidepressant and mood-regulating properties. The herb has been a remedy for symptoms linked to mild to moderate depression, anxiety, and certain mood disorders.

Scientifically, it is posited that St. John's Wort functions by enhancing the levels of specific neurotransmitters in our brain, prominently serotonin. Nevertheless, caution is urged when considering its consumption.

Potential interactions with other drugs and heightened sensitivity to sunlight are among the noted concerns, making it imperative to seek professional guidance before use.

# 50. Tulsi (Ocimum sanctum)

## Healing Properties:

Revered in Ayurveda as the "Elixir of Life", Tulsi, or Holy Basil, stands out for its adaptogenic and antimicrobial traits.

## Benefits:

Tulsi offers a multi-dimensional approach to well-being. It's not just a stress reliever but also acts as a potent immune booster. Additionally, its benefits extend to respiratory wellness, digestive support, and enhancing mental focus.

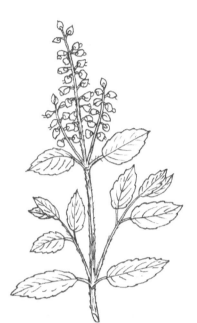

## Practical Applications:

Whether you're brewing a refreshing tea with its leaves or sprinkling them onto dishes, Tulsi is versatile. For those exploring holistic aromatherapy or seeking skin solutions, the diluted Tulsi essential oil is a must-try.

## Usage and History:

Tulsi is more than just an herb in Ayurveda; it's an emblem of sanctity and an integral part of Indian culture. With roots tracing back millennia, its reputation primarily revolves around its adaptogenic properties, providing a natural shield against stress.

But that's just scratching the surface. From clarifying the mind and fending off anxiety to reinforcing the immune defenses and ensuring a healthy digestive process, Tulsi is an all-encompassing solution for holistic health. The preferred ways to incorporate Tulsi into daily regimens are as a herbal tea or as part of Ayurvedic concoctions.

# 51. Turmeric (Curcuma longa)

## Healing Properties:

Turmeric, often referred to as the "Golden Spice," boasts potent anti-inflammatory and antioxidant capabilities, making it a staple in natural healing.

## Benefits:

Beyond just a culinary delight, Turmeric's potential benefits encompass a vast range. From nurturing joint wellness to fostering cognitive prowess and aiding the digestive process, this spice wears many hats.

## Practical Applications:

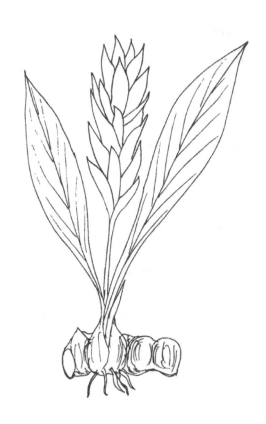

Its vibrant yellow hue can be spotted in various culinary delights, especially in Indian dishes. For a health boost, add powdered turmeric to shakes, teas, or consider supplements for a concentrated dose. If skin rejuvenation is on your radar, a turmeric paste might be your answer.

## Usage and History:

With a rich history intertwined with Indian culinary and medicinal traditions, Turmeric has graced Ayurvedic remedies for millennia. The spotlight is often on curcumin, a compound inherent to turmeric, praised for its potential health-enhancing abilities.

From pacifying inflammation and bolstering joint mobility to stimulating digestive vitality and supporting cognitive functions, Turmeric's resume is commendable. Whether it's elevating a dish's flavor or supplementing wellness routines, Turmeric remains an invaluable asset.

# 52. Valerian (Valeriana officinalis)

## Healing Properties:

Valerian, often termed "nature's valium," is lauded for its sleep-inducing and tranquilizing qualities, making it a favored natural remedy for those grappling with sleep disturbances or heightened stress.

## Benefits:

With a primary role in ushering in relaxation, Valerian elevates sleep quality and curtails anxiety bouts. Additionally, its potential in providing relief from menstrual discomfort adds to its repertoire of benefits.

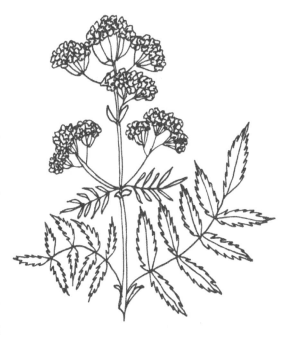

## Practical Applications:

While the Valerian root can be brewed into a tea, its distinct and somewhat overpowering flavor might not sit well with all. Therefore, encapsulated versions or tinctures are frequently opted for. When using it as a tea, pairing it with milder, pleasant-tasting herbs can mask its strong essence.

## Usage and History:

Originating in the realms of Europe and Asia, this perennial herb's legacy is deeply embedded in traditional medicinal practices, predominantly for its sleep-aid and calming capabilities. By potentially elevating gamma-aminobutyric acid (GABA) concentrations in the brain, which plays a pivotal role in inducing sleep and modulating anxiety, Valerian promotes tranquility.

Whether sipped as tea, ingested in capsules, or applied as tinctures, Valerian remains a cherished remedy in herbal pharmacopeias.

## 53.  White Willow Bark (Salix alba)

**Healing Properties:**

White Willow Bark, often dubbed "nature's aspirin," boasts potent analgesic and anti-inflammatory attributes.

**Benefits:**

Its natural composition aids in attenuating pain, curbing inflammation, providing relief from headaches, and ensuring joint comfort.

**Practical Applications:**

Traditionally consumed as a tea, White Willow Bark can also be encapsulated or transformed into tinctures. As with many natural remedies, it's essential to adhere to suggested doses.

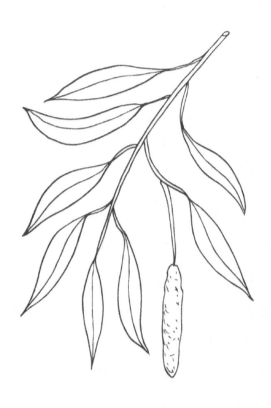

Furthermore, care should be taken to avoid extensive usage or mixing it with medications, especially those that influence blood coagulation.

**Usage and History:**

White Willow Bark traces its medicinal lineage to both European and Native American traditional healing practices. Its therapeutic prowess can be credited to salicin, a compound bearing resemblance to the active constituent in aspirin. Historically, this bark has been a remedy for diverse pain types – from headaches to musculoskeletal discomfort.

It also finds application in minimizing inflammation and managing fevers. Whether sipped in a soothing tea or taken as a supplement, White Willow Bark has cemented its place in herbal medicine.

# 54.  Wormwood (Artemisia absinthium)

**Healing Properties:**

Wormwood stands out for its potent digestive and antimicrobial attributes.

**Benefits:**

The herb's components can bolster digestion, offer relief from bloating and gas, ensure liver health, and actively counteract intestinal parasites.

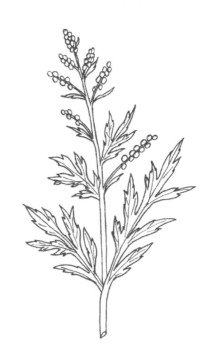

**Practical Applications:**

Wormwood's benefits are often harnessed by brewing it as tea, integrating it into digestive bitters, or by ingesting it as a supplement, either in tincture or capsule forms. It finds its prime use in addressing digestive concerns and as a countermeasure against parasitic invasions.

**Usage and History:**

Originating in regions spanning Europe, Asia, and North Africa, Wormwood has a rich history rooted in traditional medicine. Its unique properties make it a favored choice for addressing digestive perturbations such as indigestion, bloating, and suppressed appetite.

Moreover, Wormwood also carved a niche for itself in the realm of beverages with its integral role in absinthe production. A word of caution though; Wormwood harbors a chemical known as thujone which, when consumed in elevated amounts, can be toxic. As with any potent herb, prudent use under a qualified healthcare expert's supervision is recommended.

## 55. Yarrow (Achillea millefolium)

**Healing Properties:**

Yarrow stands out for its astringent and anti-inflammatory attributes, making it especially potent for accelerating wound healing and fortifying digestive health.

**Benefits:**

Among its benefits, Yarrow can staunch bleeding, enhance the wound healing process, mitigate gastrointestinal distress, and promote overall digestive health.

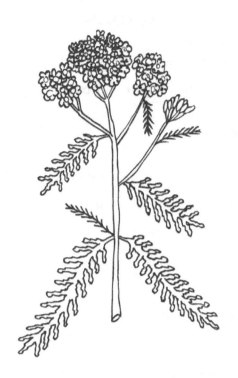

**Practical Applications:**

When it comes to practical applications, Yarrow can be applied directly to the skin as a poultice or integrated into salves tailored for wound management. For internal use, Yarrow can be brewed as a calming tea or ingested in the form of a capsule or tincture.

**Usage and History:**

Historically, Yarrow, characterized by its distinctive flowering appearance, has been embraced in traditional medicinal practices for its therapeutic attributes. Renowned for its potential in expediting wound healing and offering mild pain relief, Yarrow finds its primary use in topical applications to curb bleeding, seal wounds, and soothe skin afflictions.

Beyond these, Yarrow is credited with anti-inflammatory prowess and diuretic effects. Consuming Yarrow as a tea offers a soothing experience, while topical preparations have been longstanding remedies in herbal medicine.

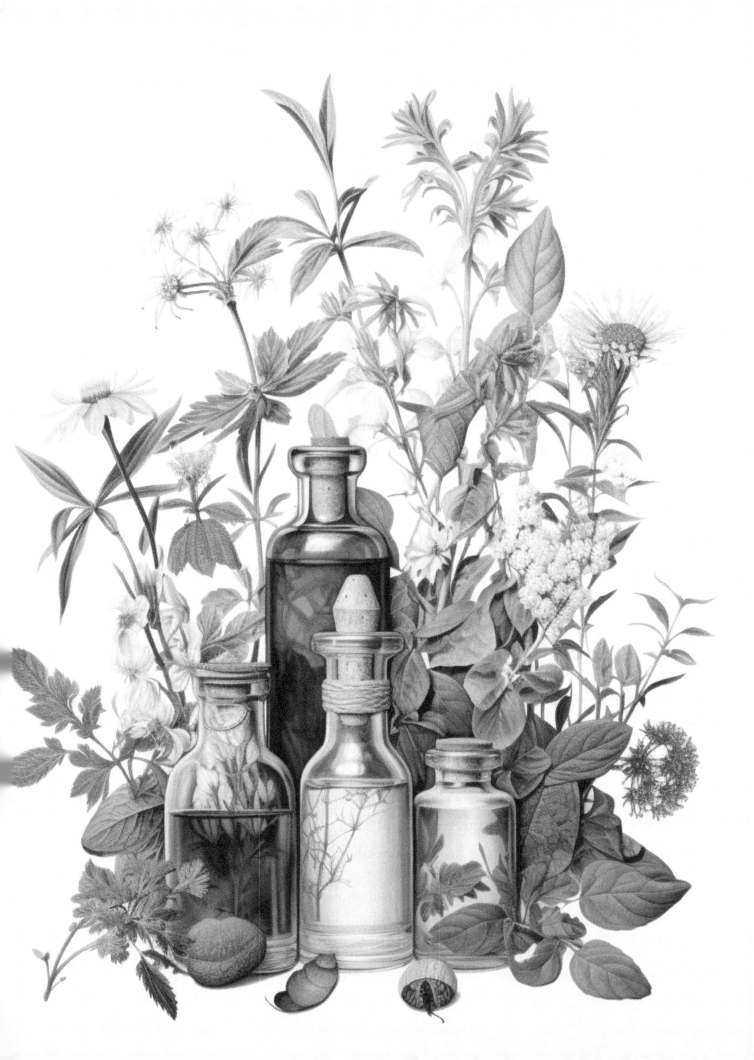

# BOOK 4: HERBAL DISPENSATORY

## Introduction

Dive into the intriguing "Herbal Dispensatory," a comprehensive resource that beckons you to delve deep into the realm of botanical remedies. This book promises a transformative journey, introducing you to nature's vast medicinal arsenal and ways to harness the power of healing herbs.

The Herbal Dispensatory stands as a testament to the timeless wisdom that's been woven into human evolution. It seamlessly blends age-old herbal traditions with contemporary scientific insights. Whether you're a seasoned practitioner or just venturing into the world of herbs, this book equips you with the knowledge to set up your herbal haven and tap into the profound benefits of natural remedies. Within these pages, you'll uncover the remarkable therapeutic properties of a myriad of herbs, each bearing its unique restorative charm.

The Herbal Dispensatory unveils the diverse and potent world of botanicals that have garnered reverence across civilizations, from common kitchen staples to rare plants from distant lands. But this book is more than just an encyclopedia of herbal remedies and culinary tips. It's an invitation to realign with the verdant world, acknowledging the deep bond we share with plants.

It champions the symbiotic relationship humans have enjoyed with flora and underscores the unparalleled healing essence nature offers. Beyond understanding the therapeutic virtues of specific plants, you'll gain insights into holistic health. This book introduces you to the principles of herbal dynamics, energetics, and personalized herbal strategies, enabling you to craft tailored herbal solutions for individual needs.

By turning to the wisdom encapsulated in the Herbal Dispensatory, we're invited to transition from the bustling realm of artificial medications to the serene yet potent curative treasures nature bestows. It's an opportunity to nurture a profound bond with our planet, realizing that it generously provides everything essential for our health and vitality.

Let the Herbal Dispensatory be your steadfast companion on this enlightening journey. Immerse yourself in the mystique and knowledge of botanical healing, cultivate medicinal plants, and tap into the benevolent gifts nature freely extends. May this guide embolden and steer you as you weave the therapeutic essence of herbs into your daily life. Let it kindle a passion for practicing herbalism autonomously, fostering wellness, vitality, and a renewed bond with nature. Embark on this enchanting voyage today.

# Chapter 1: Growing Medicinal Plants

## Choose the Right Location

- **Sunlight Evaluation:** Medicinal plants come with a spectrum of sunlight needs, from craving continuous sun to preferring dappled shade. Grasp the need to pinpoint each plant's sunlight requirement and scrutinize your garden's daily sunlight patterns. Understand methods to enhance sunlight or create shade based on the preferences of your herbs.

- **Analyzing Soil and Drainage:** The health of your medicinal flora hinges on the soil's texture and make-up. Delve into the necessity of a soil examination to measure its pH balance and nutrient profile. Discover how to enrich the soil with organic components, optimizing drainage and fertility for your herbaceous haven. Acknowledge the need for good drainage to stave off excess water and root decay.

- **Spotting Microclimates and Niches:** Gardens can harbor distinct microclimates and niches—localized environmental conditions contrasting with the broader regional climate. Learn to pinpoint these unique zones in your garden, like sun-drenched patches by a barrier or shaded spots beneath trees. Recognize the advantage of using these zones by planting herbs attuned to particular thermal and humidity conditions.

- **Considering Wind and Ventilation:** Reflect on the influence of wind patterns and air movement on your herbs. While light breezes aid in spreading pollen and thwarting diseases, harsh gusts can harm fragile plants. Delve into strategies to erect wind barriers, like putting up shrubs or introducing robust companion flora, shielding your plants from harsh wind.

- **Ease of Access and Practicality:** When earmarking a spot for your herbal garden, prioritize its accessibility and practicality. Opt for a locale that's within easy reach for routine care, plucking, and upkeep. Contemplate factors such as closeness to water, unobstructed pathways, and the overall ease in managing your botanicals.

- **Environmental Awareness:** Factor in external environmental aspects that could affect your garden, like nearby pollutants, adjacent pesticide application, or chemical seepage risks. Pinpoint a spot that cuts down contamination threats, fostering the emergence of pure, vigorous medicinal plants.

By meticulously weighing these elements when pinpointing your garden's locale, you're laying the groundwork for fruitful cultivation and ample harvests. Keep in mind, each botanical has its distinct needs, so invest in understanding the specifics of your chosen plants. With the right spot, you're ensuring a setting where your medicinal flora thrives, gifting you with a robust and continuous supply of curative botanical wonders.

As you set forth on your herbal cultivation voyage, the Herbal Dispensatory is your go-to reference, brimming with actionable insights, recommendations, and encouragement to help you shape your herbal oasis. Relish the delight of caring for these incredible botanicals, watching them evolve from mere seeds into mighty curatives, ready to rejuvenate your health and spirit.

## Difference in Growing Herbs Indoors and Outdoors

Based on your convenience, you can grow herbs either indoors or outdoors. Regardless of the setting, herbs thrive in well-draining soil, stable temperatures, and adequate sunlight. This applies whether you're placing them on a windowsill or in an outdoor garden. Though the choice of where to establish your herb garden ultimately rests with you, it's worth noting that some herbs naturally fare better outside than inside.

The following is a list of herbs that can be grown inside:

- Sage
- Anise
- Amaranth
- Angelica

- Ashwagandha
- Balsam Fir
- Lemon Balm
- Basil

If you like to plant in the open air, go for these outdoor herbs:

- Rosemary
- Agave
- Parsley
- Aloe

- Coriander
- Balsam Root
- Mint
- Chives

## Growing Indoors

Growing herbs can be an ideal pastime, especially if you're confined at home and are keen to pick up a new hobby. Whether indoors or outdoors, herbs are easy to cultivate, wallet-friendly, and offer a delightful activity for both adults and kids. The bonus? Freshly picked rosemary or basil can elevate any meal, from pastas to roasted dishes.

Starting an herb garden is straightforward. With the right tools, pots, and a game plan, you're good to go. Here's a step-by-step guide to get you started:

**Step 1: Picking the Right Pot**

Having a home herb garden offers the luxury of easy access. Need a sprinkle of flavor for your dishes? Grab some fresh basil, thyme, or sage. Select a pot and position it in a suitable spot, be it your patio, balcony, or kitchen. The challenge often lies in selecting the right pot. With myriad options, like wood, clay, resin, and metal, it's crucial to prioritize drainage. Ensure your chosen pot has drainage holes. Mason jars might look chic but don't bode well for herbs due to the lack of drainage, risking root rot. Also, size matters. An overly spacious pot can cause your plants to focus on root growth, while a cramped one can restrict growth. Opt for a pot that strikes a balance.

## Step 2: Deciding on Your Herbs

For first-timers, it's best to stick to the classics. Mint, basil, and parsley are great beginner plants; they grow quickly and are hardy. Here's a quick rundown on a few favorites:

• **Basil**: Loves the sun and is low-maintenance. Keep the soil moist and well-drained.

• **Mint**: Perfect for pots given its tendency to spread. It can handle shade but loves direct sun.

• **Oregano**: Packed with flavor in its tiny leaves. It craves sunlight and well-drained soil. Greek oregano, especially, should be kept indoors during colder months.

• **Parsley**: Chefs' favorite, the flat-leaf variety, has a robust flavor. It thrives in damp, well-drained soil and can handle a bit of shade.

• **Thyme**: Known for its aroma, it loves dry conditions, direct sun, and well-draining soil.

• **Rosemary**: A fragrant herb that prefers cooler climates, abundant light, and slightly moist soil. Consider moving it indoors during winter.

## Step 3: Opt for Starters Over Seeds

For beginners, it's advisable to begin with young plants instead of seeds. This fast-tracks your growth by several weeks and increases the odds of a bountiful yield.

## Step 4: Choosing the Right Soil

When potting, favor potting mix over garden soil. The former offers better drainage while the latter can hold excess moisture in containers. A garden trowel will also come in handy for various tasks like digging and weeding.

## Step 5: Harvesting and Care

Tending and Harvesting Herbs, like all plants, need consistent care. Regular watering is crucial, and frequent pruning can stimulate new growth. Remember, each herb has specific care requirements, so harvest accordingly.

## Growing Outdoors

Starting an outdoor herb garden largely mirrors the steps involved in pot cultivation. The primary advantage outdoors is the natural soil. However, it's essential to prepare the ground correctly to get the best from your herbs. Here's a streamlined guide to setting up an outdoor herb garden:

**Step 1: Assess Soil Quality** Herbs prefer less fertile soil. A professional soil test can gauge its nutrient levels, helping you decide if any fertilization is needed. Over-fertilizing can dilute the herbs' aroma, flavor, and medicinal properties. The only exceptions are herbs grown for their flowers, which may require richer soil for optimal growth.

**Step 2: Prep the Planting Site** Choose your garden spot, then dig small planting holes, keeping enough space between each. Even if space is at a premium, herbs don't need much room to flourish.

**Step 3: Plant with Care** Before placing your herbs in the holes, gently loosen the roots to promote better soil integration. Cover the roots with soil, leaving the plant exposed to soak up the sun. Adequate sunlight is crucial for herbs, influencing their taste, aroma, and essential oil production.

**Step 4: Maintain Moisture Levels** Consistently monitor the soil's moisture. While some herbs like thyme, lavender, and rosemary tolerate drier conditions, they still need periodic watering. Avoid both underwatering and overwatering. Overly wet soil can harm some herbs, especially if you intend to use the roots.

**Step 5: Harvest and Prune** Regular harvesting or pruning can keep your garden tidy and encourage plant growth. Without it, some herbs may become leggy or start seeding prematurely. For perennial herbs like lavender, sage, and rosemary, pruning can lead to bushier growth. Typically, it's safe to trim up to 2/3 of perennial herbs at season's end. Some, like rosemary and lavender, can even be pruned back severely once they've established a robust root system.

In summary, while outdoor herb gardening requires effort, the rewards are bountiful. Whether you choose to garden directly in the soil or prefer pots placed outdoors, ensure that you cater to the specific needs of each herb. Over time, you'll cultivate not only a garden but also a keen understanding of these aromatic plants.

## Safety Tips for Gardening

Before cultivating medicinal plants, it's vital to understand the necessary precautions and potential interactions. Some herbs can interfere with how the body processes prescription drugs, and others might be unsuitable for certain health issues.

Ensure you consult an expert and gather comprehensive information on the herbs you aim to plant. Your medicinal garden will generally repel pests due to the potent scents of the herbs. To further deter pests, consider using herbs as companion plants. Delve into research to find optimal methods for safeguarding your garden against pests and diseases.

For variety, consider rotating the planting spots for annual herbs. Introduce compost and organic waste to encourage the growth of helpful organisms. Regularly maintain your garden: weed, nourish, hydrate, and mulch your plants, ensuring the surroundings remain free from weeds. Lastly, familiarize yourself with beneficial insects to prevent mistakenly eliminating them from your garden.

## Essential Tools

For a successful herb garden, ensure you have these essential tools:

- A long-handled shovel to facilitate planting, especially when you're introducing a variety of herbs.
- A pointed digging instrument for hard-to-access spots, especially if your primary shovel isn't long enough.
- A watering can accompanied by a moisture gauge to monitor and maintain the right hydration levels.
- An aesthetically pleasing pot or container for your seeds or soil. Ideally, maintain about an inch of soil over the root system, aiding their growth.
- A bag of compost-rich soil. Opt for a dark soil mixture that includes peat moss and added nutrients for enhanced plant growth.

## Organic vs. Non-Organic

When nurturing your garden, be cautious about the choice of fertilizers and pesticides. Opt for organic seeds and plant them in chemical-free soil. Growing plants indoors may reduce the need for organic methods. Yet, outdoor spaces like balconies or sunny windowsills are also suitable but come with risks like cold exposure. To safeguard your plants, it's essential to study the specific needs of the herbs you're growing.

**Garden Essentials**

Your garden should ideally possess these qualities:

• Be devoid of weeds.

• Receive ample sunlight.

• Be well-tended and enriched with organic manure.

• Consistently watered throughout summer without making the soil too soggy.

• Avoid excessively damp or hot soil conditions to prevent diseases or potential plant death.

Proper soil treatment is the foundation of healthy plant growth. However, a common oversight is not understanding the compatibility of certain herbs with one's local climate and conditions. Initiating a home apothecary should begin with your garden, which can then act as a resource during health emergencies.

Usually, July and August are ideal for herb harvesting, as post-summer, many enter a dormant phase, becoming tough and dry. This period is also prime for herb processing into medicinal forms. Moreover, a home apothecary is a fantastic platform to enlighten loved ones about the benefits of natural remedies.

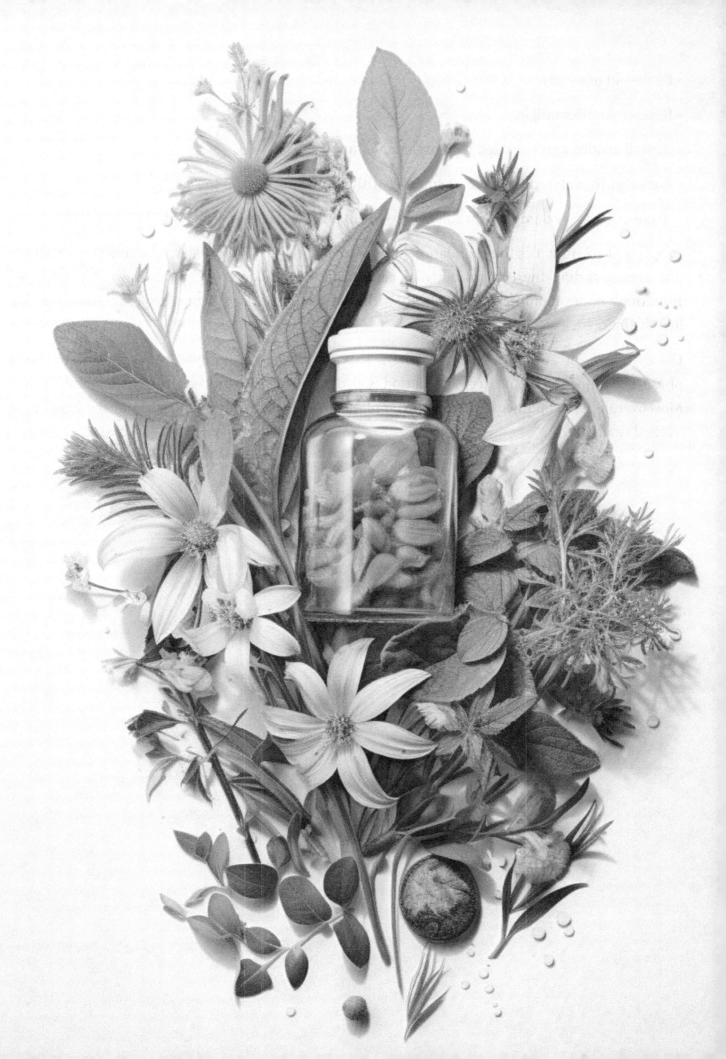

# BOOK 5: NATURAL HERBAL ANTIBIOTICS

## Introduction

Step into the fascinating domain of "Natural Herbal Antibiotics." This tome unravels the extraordinary capabilities of plants in managing infections and boosting our innate healing prowess. Herein, you'll embark on a journey to unearth nature's treasure trove of powerful antimicrobial agents and their role in holistic health. In an era marked by growing antibiotic resistance, the search for safe and effective alternatives has never been more pressing.

This manuscript acts as a beacon, shedding light on herbal antibiotics, underscoring their ancient use, empirical evidence, and relevance in today's world. Drawing from the collective wisdom of herbalists, healers, and age-old medicinal practices, "Natural Herbal Antibiotics" dives deep into the traditions and medical systems from various corners of the world.

By marrying this age-old wisdom with contemporary research, we glean into plants' immense curative powers against formidable infections.

- **The Global Health Challenge:** Grasp the magnitude of the health crisis triggered by antibiotic resistance. Delve into its root causes and the dire need for alternative healing. Uncover how herbal antibiotics emerge as a promising and efficacious response to this looming concern.

- **Herbal Science Demystified:** Navigate the scientific principles behind the antimicrobial prowess of plants. Delve into the bioactive compounds within herbs that battle bacteria, viruses, fungi, and parasites. Unravel their modus operandi in supporting our immune defenses.

- **Harnessing Herbal Power:** Dive into a diverse array of herbal antibiotics, each boasting unique antibacterial spectra. Explore their traditional uses, dosage guidelines, and effective preparation methods. This volume highlights an array of potent natural remedies, from renowned ones like berberine-centric herbs and essential oils to the less-charted territories of Echinacea, oregano, and garlic.

- **Woven into Daily Life**: Learn the art of seamlessly integrating herbal antibiotics into your daily regime, be it for acute care or preventive strategies. Delve into holistic immune boosters, stress alleviation methods, and dietary shifts. Master the craft of concocting personalized herbal blends by synergistically combining plants.

Dive deep into "Natural Herbal Antibiotics" and uncover the myriad antibacterial wonders nature presents. Empower yourself with knowledge, enabling informed choices for your holistic well-being. Embrace a therapeutic paradigm that melds time-honored traditions with cutting-edge research.

Join us on this enlightening voyage through the universe of herbal antibiotics. Reestablish the age-old bond between humans and flora, nurturing a profound bond with Earth and tapping into nature's bounty for our health and vigor. Let this book be your trusted compass, guiding you towards a brighter, sustainable tomorrow.

# Chapter 1: Harvesting & Processing

## Herbal Preparation

Understanding the characteristics of herbs is essential before delving into their applications. Herbs offer diverse uses, ranging from culinary to medicinal. Over time, various techniques for crafting herbal solutions have evolved, each offering distinct advantages and disadvantages. These methods, polished over generations, hinge on the understanding that different parts of a plant possess varied healing properties with varying strengths. For example, while some herbs infuse well into oils, others are more suited for tinctures.

Before venturing into making personal herbal concoctions, thorough research is a must. While resources like this book provide a foundation, it's crucial to delve deeper to prevent undesirable mixtures. Visiting local herb shops can give insights into herb packaging and dosages. Familiarize yourself with a herb's strength and effects, and avoid those you're unsure of. Moreover, recognizing which part of the plant you're using - be it leaves, roots, or stems - is crucial as each carries distinct properties.

As a guideline, typically one ounce of a herb or a blend suffices. You'd typically need fewer fresh herbs than dried. Consider cultivating herbs or foraging them, but exercise caution in the latter to avoid potentially harmful plants. The key is to apply herbs as directly as possible to the area needing treatment. For instance, instead of drinking tea for a foot splinter, you'd directly remove it.

Herbal remedies work over time, unlike instant results from prescriptions. They operate gradually, necessitating continuous use to witness changes. These changes vary per individual, and their effectiveness is gauged by their ability to restore the body's natural balance. Chronic issues might require prolonged herbal treatments. If you've endured a problem for years, expect many months of herbal treatments for resolution.

When crafting herbal remedies, it's advisable to refresh them daily and keep preparations simple. Proper measurements are pivotal to ensure safety. Despite being 'natural', herbs require caution in usage. Overconsumption can be detrimental, emphasizing the need for patience and correct dosages.

It's imperative to avoid aluminum utensils for herbal preparations and, given the vast array of medicinal herbs, it's natural to feel daunted initially by the choices and processes involved.

After grasping the essence of herbs, the subsequent move is to discover their application in herbal solutions. Herbs serve multiple purposes, from medicines to culinary delights. Crafting herbal remedies involves varied techniques, each boasting its pros and cons. Historically, these methods have been fine-tuned over ages for health benefits.

It's common knowledge among herbalists that different plant parts hold specific healing qualities with varied intensities. Some plants excel when infused in oils, while others shine in tinctures and elixirs. The preparation method directly influences the remedy's strength.

Prior to crafting herbal solutions, comprehensive research is vital. While this text offers foundational knowledge, further exploration is needed to sidestep incompatible herb mixtures. Perfecting the art of herbal remedies demands patience and experimentation.

In addition to online resources, local herb stores or health shops are great places to understand herb packaging. Often, herbs with alike traits are grouped together. Labels also provide dosage guidelines, which should be strictly followed. Always acquaint yourself with an herb's properties before using it, especially unfamiliar ones.

The specific plant part utilized plays a role. From leaves, roots, and stems to seeds and flowers, each segment has distinct effects, necessitating dosage adjustments. A general guideline suggests using one ounce of an individual or mixed herb. Opt for fewer fresh herbs over dried ones. Whether you use dried or fresh herbs, cultivating your own is cost-effective if space permits. With keen observation, you can even harvest wild herbs. Yet, caution is paramount. Mistaking harmful plants for benign ones, like confusing deadly nightshade for jimson weed, can be perilous. If in doubt, source herbs from reputable stores.

When contemplating the best herbal preparation, the aim is efficient delivery to the affected body part. For example, for a foot splinter, you wouldn't drink tea hoping for it to eject; you'd extract it manually. The same logic applies to herbs. A headache might benefit from a direct poultice application to the forehead.

Understand that herbal solutions don't provide instant relief like most medications. Their effect is gradual and consistent application yields results. If opting for teas, consume consistently till there's improvement, usually within three days. Effectiveness varies per individual.

The merit of herbs lies in their ability to naturally recalibrate the body. Instant long-term benefits from a single dose are rare. Persistent intake usually brings lasting results. For chronic ailments, the rule of thumb is a month of herbal intake for each year of ailment duration.

Always opt for fresh preparations when using medicinal herbs. These can be stored for long if done correctly. It's wise to start simple, mastering single herbs before venturing into blends. Due to diverse preparation methods, accurate measurements are essential to avoid adverse effects.

Aim for long-term holistic health when crafting remedies. While powerful, herbs demand caution. Unlike prescribed medicines with immediate results, herbs work over time. Hastiness and overconsumption can backfire. The misconception that 'natural' equates to 'safe' can be misleading.

Lastly, steer clear of aluminum cookware for herbal preparations. The vastness of the herbal world can be daunting, given the plethora of herbs and preparation techniques.

## Drying Herbs

If you don't dry and store your herbs appropriately, their potency will diminish rapidly. Fresh herbs lose their strength quickly, so it's ideal to dry them immediately if they aren't going to be used soon.

To dry them, detach the leaves from the stems and lay them flat on a clean surface. Bigger plants can be suspended in a dry spot, like a heated basement or loft. If insects are drawn to them, cover the herbs with a light cloth.

How long it takes for an herb to dry depends on the type of herb and the drying method. It's preferable to dry them swiftly, as prolonged drying can reduce their efficacy.

Typically, it takes about a week for most herbs to dry. An herb is sufficiently dried if it's aromatic yet snaps easily. If it crumbles entirely upon touch, it's been dried too much. Roots need a longer drying time, usually more than three weeks, and they should be cleaned beforehand.

While old images may show herbs dangling in older homes, today we have better storage methods. Herbs stored in sealed glass jars can last up to five years, while tinctures in similar containers can last a decade. However, oils and balms, which can become stale, typically last between six months to a year.

Drying has been a longstanding preservation technique, even among Native Americans. They used sun drying and salt curing to dry berries, roots, and meats. Dried herbs often went into broths, and dried berries were baked in pies. Mixing dried foods with sweeteners like honey or maple syrup made for tasty snacks. These dried items are nutrient-rich, packed with vitamin C and protein.

There are multiple methods to dry herbs, fruits, and vegetables. They were often dried wrapped in leaves or wooden pieces. The ideal drying location is airy and shaded. It's helpful to know which plants dry best under sunlight.

Here's what you need to know about drying different parts of plants:

- **Leaves and Flowers:** These shouldn't be washed. Just shake off any dirt or bugs. If the stems are minimal, group them into bundles. Or you can lay them flat on surfaces like screens to dry.

- **Barks:** If needed, scrape off the bark, a process known as tossing.

- **Roots:** They can be bundled together or spread out. Usually, rinsing is enough to clean off soil, but for roots with clay, you might need a hose and some manual scrubbing. Large, non-aromatic roots can be split down the center.

To ensure complete drying, plant parts should be brittle to touch. For hanging plants, it's advisable to trim the bottommost leaves. For a large root, split it to check if the center is dry.

## Storing Herbs

Avoid exposing your herbs to light or extreme heat to maintain their aroma and essential properties. Before storing herbs, make sure that containers like food-grade fiber barrels and plastic bags are entirely dry. Label them with the date and where they were sourced.

Crushed or processed herbs tend to lose their potency quicker than whole ones. Here are some general guidelines for preserving fresh herbs:

• Fresh herbs can typically remain vibrant for 4-6 weeks with proper care, but under optimal storage conditions, they might last up to a year.

• Try to avoid using plastic containers for herbs. If you must use plastic, glass or sturdy freezer bags are better choices. Some plastics can emit chemicals that negatively affect the herbs, even in a fridge.

• Storing herbs in a cool, shaded area prolongs their shelf life.

• If herbs come in plastic bags, retain them in their original packaging for easier identification during culinary tasks.

• Freezing is a useful method to store herbs. Most herbs can retain their taste for up to six months when frozen.

• To protect the herbs' aromatic and essential properties, keep them away from direct sunlight and heat. Ensure that herbs are thoroughly dry before storing them in food-grade bags or containers that are airtight.

• Broken or crushed herbs degrade faster than whole herbs.

Remember, herbs typically have a short lifespan. Even the best storage methods might not prolong their freshness as much as hoped, especially if you're working with fresh instead of dried varieties. While herbs play a vital role in health treatments, don't hesitate to use them generously. The storage conditions might seem within your control, but factors like humidity, $CO_2$, oxygen, and ethylene levels might not always be manageable. With various items in a fridge, maintaining a consistent temperature might be challenging. Instead of chasing perfection, focus on spotting and resolving potential issues.

While refrigerating herbs is an option, it can be space-consuming, and there's a risk of spilling contents. Dried herbs offer a storage advantage. You can crush them into various forms, like powders or dried leaves, and store them in labeled airtight containers. Since fresh herbs degrade swiftly, many prefer to dry them. Typically, they need about a week to dry. Roots, after thorough washing, take about three weeks longer than leaves and flowers. An herb is deemed dry when it's still somewhat aromatic but can be snapped. If it turns to dust upon touch, it's over-dried.

To dry herbs, detach the leaves from stems and lay them in loose layers on a clean surface. Plastic bags or containers are not ideal for storage as they might absorb the herbs' essential oils. Opt for containers like glazed ceramic, dark glass, or metal with secure lids for storing completely dried herbs.

For bigger plants, hang them in dry spots like a warm basement or loft. To shield them from pests, drape them in cheesecloth.

Transparent glass jars are suitable for herb storage as they allow easy monitoring for any spoilage signs. Store these jars in a dark area, possibly shielded by curtains or doors.

## Wildcrafting

Wildcrafting refers to the practice of collecting plants from their natural habitats. Often linked to Native Americans who adapted to the nuances of their environment, this type of herbalism has deep roots in ancient traditions.

Wildcrafting primarily involves harvesting seeds and berries from the wild, serving both nutritional and medicinal needs. It was the Native Americans who popularized this method, relying on it for sustenance and healing.

The art of wildcrafting can be intricate. It often involves navigating deep into untouched terrains like dense forests or remote hillsides, away from common pathways and human activity. Knowledge of the native flora is essential for foragers, as there's a risk of encountering toxic plants. Proper identification and understanding of each plant and its components are paramount before any harvesting can take place.

Many enthusiasts keen on wildcrafting venture into their local wilds, explore diverse landscapes, or even inspect their own backyards. This hands-on approach helps familiarize them with potential medicinal plants in the vicinity. To the surprise of many newcomers, the art of wildcrafting is often more accessible than presumed, thanks to various resources like regional herb maps.

In contemporary times, wildcrafting has seen a resurgence in interest, particularly among groups like Wiccans or Pagans who have a penchant for herbology.

Like all natural resources, herbs need careful and sustainable harvesting to prevent over-exploitation. A principled wildcrafter will always ensure that neither nature nor fellow humans are harmed, reflecting values deeply embedded in Native American traditions.

Observing a plant's natural habitat is vital. This includes noting neighboring flora, the insects it attracts, the nature of the soil, sunlight exposure, and proximity to water sources. Even with limited knowledge about a plant, its environment can offer significant insights.

## Harvesting

When harvesting herbs, the goal is to capture them when their aromatic oils, which contribute to their flavor and aroma, are at their zenith. To harvest effectively, it's crucial to understand the specific uses of the herb. For instance, herbs cultivated primarily for their leaves should be gathered before they bloom. Although chive flowers can be visually appealing, the act of flowering alters the leaf's taste. Thus, if the foliage is the desired part, chives should be picked before flowering.

For herbs grown for their seeds, the ideal time to harvest is when the seed pods transition from green to brown or gray. However, it's essential to gather them before the pods burst open. Herb flowers, like chamomile and borage, are best collected right before they fully bloom. Herbs with valuable roots, such as goldenseal, ginseng, and chicory, should ideally be harvested in the fall, after they've shed their leaves.

Here are some general harvesting guidelines for herbs:

1. **Harvest Timing:** Begin harvesting when the plant has enough foliage to continue growing. At one time, you can harvest up to 75% of a season's growth.

2. **Best Time of Day:** Harvest early in the day after the dew has dried but before the sun gets too hot.

3. **Flowering:** If you're growing an herb for its leaves, harvest before it flowers, as flowering can inhibit leaf production.

4. **Flower Buds:** Harvest just after flower buds appear but before they open to capture the maximum flavor and oil concentration.

5. **Annual Herbs:** These can be harvested up until the frost.

6. **Perennial Herbs:** These should be harvested until late August, ceasing about a month before the first frost.

When harvesting different parts of herbal plants, here's a brief guide:

- **Flowers:** Harvest after the first bloom, using shears or a tool that gathers multiple flower stalks together.

- **Mushrooms:** Gently twist the mushroom base counterclockwise to avoid bruising.

- **Roots:** Use a garden tool to gently extract the roots from the ground. Clean them off afterwards.

- **Bark:** Use a knife to carefully remove bark from branches.

- **Berries:** Pick directly from the plant and wash before use.

- **Buds:** These can be gently picked or removed using a specific harvesting tool. Always dry immediately.

- **Leaves:** Pluck directly or use a leaf-stripping tool for efficiency.

- **Whole Plant:** Use a knife to cleanly cut, keeping in mind the type of plant (annual or perennial) to ensure the proper method is used.

- **Aerial Parts:** Cut the stem above the lowest leaf set, then separate and spread the leaves to dry.

- **Flowering Tops:** Cut and place in water. Remove leaves from submerged stems.

In summary, the harvesting process for herbs requires knowledge and precision to maximize the efficacy and benefits of the plant parts. Proper harvesting ensures the best quality for medicinal or culinary uses.

# Chapter 2: How to Use Herbs Safely

For those venturing into the realm of herbal remedies for the first time, several questions may arise: Which herbs should one choose? When is the right time to consume them? How can one determine the right herb for their specific needs or ailments? Delving into the wisdom of Native Americans can shed light on these questions, as they have harnessed the power of plants for healing for countless generations.

Native Americans approached plants with a reverence and understanding, akin to the way we rely on prescription medicines today. Depending on the specific illness or ailment, they would turn to different plants for remedies, though they always followed certain fundamental principles.

The indigenous peoples have always been open to sharing their deep-seated knowledge, welcoming those who approach them with sincerity and gratitude. It's essential to note that, much like modern medications or substances like alcohol, herbs too can be detrimental if misused. For Native Americans, everything in existence—from minerals to plants, animals to humans—had a designated purpose and role in the grand tapestry of life.

They were also cognizant of individual gastrointestinal sensitivities and could discern which herb would align best with an individual's unique constitution. Unlike the Western perspective that largely sees humans as a homogenous group with minor differences, indigenous wisdom acknowledged significant variances. For instance, someone with a naturally warmer constitution might not consume as much food or drink as another individual with a cooler disposition. Through a more holistic viewpoint, herbs are seen as an integral part of our surroundings, deserving respect and understanding, rather than apprehension.

As we delve deeper into the specific herbal practices of Native Americans, it's vital to acknowledge that the information is rooted in a blend of disciplines. Our insights are derived from a combination of anthropological, botanical, ethnobotanical, and pharmacological studies.

## Guidelines for Safe Herbal Usage

1. Ensure the plant you're considering for consumption is non-toxic to humans.
2. Recognize that certain plants can interfere with prescribed medications, leading to potential overdoses.
3. If you're prone to allergies (whether to flora, fauna, or mold), always exercise caution before trying a new herbal remedy.
4. Never impulsively consume plants from public spaces or personal gardens without adequate prior knowledge.

5. Seek information from trusted and credible resources.

6. Double-check to ensure you have identified the correct plant.

7. Opt for dried herbs as they generally have a reduced concentration of active compounds compared to their fresh counterparts.

8. Always be conscious of dosage recommendations, as the strength of herbs can differ.

9. Always avoid confusing toxic plants with those that merely resemble them but are safe.

10. Understand the distinction between wild-grown plants and those cultivated for consumption.

11. Steer clear of experimenting with unfamiliar herbs or those you can't ascertain as safe.

12. Some plants can release harmful substances when altered (like crushed or chewed), so be aware of preparation methods.

13. When introducing someone to a new herb, guide them through the safe preparation process.

14. Abstain from consuming any plant or natural substance deemed illegal in certain regions, even if used in moderation.

15. Acknowledge that indigenous communities have utilized herbs safely for generations, indicating that with proper knowledge, it can be both beneficial and safe.

## Safe Practices in Herbal Usage

When engaging with Native American herbs, or herbs from any culture for that matter, safety should always be at the forefront of one's mind. Here's a breakdown of important points from the information provided:

1. **Regulations and Authenticity**: In the U.S., plants are not held to the same stringent regulations as pharmaceutical drugs. This means that anyone can collect and sell herbs. This lack of regulation can lead to inconsistencies in potency and purity.

2. **Sourcing Herbs**: It's crucial to source your herbs from trusted suppliers. The commercial collection of certain species might be prohibited, or these plants might be protected under specific laws, requiring permits to harvest. Therefore, always check the regulations of your local area before attempting to collect any herbs.

3. **Cultural Respect**: Engaging with indigenous communities can offer authentic knowledge about traditional herbal uses. When sourcing herbs from such communities, it's essential to approach with respect, understanding that certain herbs hold significant spiritual or cultural values. Always consult local experts, such as medicine men or elders, to ensure you're using the herbs appropriately.

4. **The Risk of Abuse**: Just like any substance, there's potential for misuse and abuse. Certain herbs can be addictive, leading individuals down a path of increased tolerance, dependence, and, eventually, withdrawal. Recognizing the signs of substance abuse is crucial, whether it involves traditional herbs, alcohol, or more commonly recognized illicit drugs.

5. **Herbal Potency and Effects**: Not every herb will work as one might expect. Their effects can be subtle or may not align with one's expectations. For instance, a strong tincture might not necessarily help with emotional pain, even if it has other beneficial properties. Additionally, the environment plays a vital role in the growth and potency of herbs, meaning their effects can vary based on where and how they're sourced.

6. **Potential Dangers**: Just because a substance is natural doesn't mean it's safe. Many natural substances can be harmful or even deadly if misused. Always approach herbal remedies with the same caution you would any other medication.

In conclusion, while herbs offer a plethora of potential benefits, they also come with risks. Educate yourself, source responsibly, respect cultural significance, and always prioritize safety when experimenting with or using herbal remedies.

## Safety Tips on the Abuse of Herbs

The misuse of herbs among Native Americans has been well-documented across various studies. This practice isn't exclusive to one culture; many societies have consumed these substances historically. Overconsumption or using herbs recreationally to alter one's state of mind is what constitutes misuse. While these herbs have historical medicinal significance, their safety for modern populations hasn't been thoroughly examined.

In numerous tribes, the exploitation of herbs was widespread. They served various purposes, from therapeutic remedies during challenging times to aesthetic applications, especially for women who lacked societal platforms to accentuate their beauty. Some believed in the mystical properties of the "black drink," thinking it could alleviate fatigue, mitigate pain, and amplify strength.

Research indicates that these herbs were primarily consumed for their mood-enhancing effects. Many believed that consuming them could bridge the gap between the material and spiritual worlds. This interplay between humans and the spiritual realm has historical roots across various cultures, underlining the importance of understanding this dynamic.

The perception of these herbs was deeply rooted in spirituality. In many tribes, a dichotomy existed between those overseeing the herb's distribution and those influencing the tribe's significant decisions. These decision-makers drew insights from their experiences with the herbs, believing it enhanced their connection with the spiritual entities, which in turn guided their choices for the tribe's welfare.

For certain tribes, these herbs were deemed divine gifts, used for healing purposes. Typically, the medicine man was the primary consumer, indicating his unique spiritual bond. This consumption reinforced the belief among followers that the herbs facilitated communication with the spiritual domain.

The implications of these findings are broader than the Native American context. Beyond the individual risks posed by herbal drugs, they can also endanger those around the user. Thus, research must persistently delve into understanding the varied impacts of these herbs and their long-term health consequences.

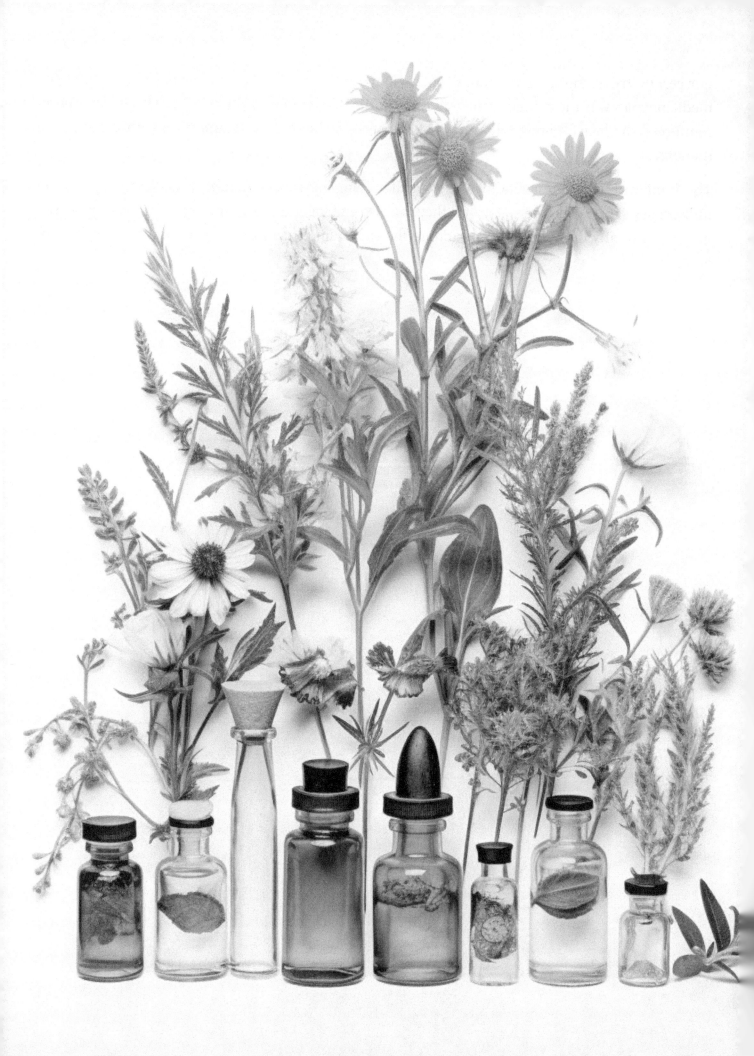

# BOOK 6: HERBAL TINCTURES AND SALVES

## Introduction

Welcome to the captivating realm of herbal tinctures and salves, a universe where botanical wonders transform into potent remedies. This book serves as your gateway into the dual spheres of the craft and knowledge of formulating herbal solutions that rejuvenate and heal. From vibrant tinctures embodying the heart of flora to comforting salves that mend the skin, we traverse the age-old legacy of unlocking the curative might of herbs.

The legacy of herbal tinctures and salves dates back eons. Civilizations, old and new, have vouched for the remedial prowess of plants and their role in bolstering health. We honor this enduring knowledge, steering you through the alchemy of conjuring your very own herbal essences and balms, thus granting access to the curative marvels of the plant kingdom.

We commence with an in-depth look at the bedrock of herbal therapeutics, acquainting you with the symbiosis of flora and health. You'll gain insights into the parts of plants vital for concoctions, their vital components, and the unique health benefits they bestow.

Following this, we demystify the craft of tincture formulation. We navigate you through the meticulous steps of harnessing plants' medicinal virtues using alcohol or glycerin, yielding powerful herbal concoctions seamlessly integrated by the body. This section enlightens you about prime herbs for tincturing, accurate dosage estimations, and conservation methods to ensure your creations retain their potency.

Subsequently, we voyage into the salve sphere, topical balms laden with herbal blessings that rejuvenate and shield the skin, directly delivering the plants' remedial attributes where needed. We shed light on diverse salve-making techniques, spanning from herb-infused oils to the amalgamation of beeswax and organic elements, achieving the ideal salve consistency.

A recurrent theme throughout the guide is the essence of procuring premium herbs and adopting eco-friendly methodologies, underscoring the reverence for Mother Earth and her botanical gifts. We touch upon moral harvesting, propelling you towards a symbiotic bond with nature as you amass and nurture your herbal companions.

Furthermore, we delve into the versatile uses of herbal tinctures and salves, addressing a spectrum of health concerns, from common colds and gut health to skin care, and beyond. We furnish an assortment of recipes, nudging you towards weaving these herbal wonders into your routine.

As you embark on this botanical voyage, bear in mind that these remedies augment, but don't substitute, expert medical advice. Collaboration with healthcare professionals is advocated, turning to them when necessary.

Our ambition is for this tome to bestow upon you the tools and confidence to morph into a proficient herbal artisan, adept at crafting tinctures and salves. By immersing in the plant realm's sagacity and harnessing the magic of herbal curatives, we envision a profound bond with nature and an invigorated health paradigm for you.

So, accompany us on this fragrant and therapeutic exploration into the universe of herbal tinctures and salves. Let this book be your beacon, acquainting you with the herbal artistry and kindling a passion for the restorative essence of our natural environment.

# Chapter 1: Recipes and Remedies

## 1. Abscess

An abscess refers to a concentrated accumulation of pus within the body's tissues due to infection or inflammation. It often presents as a raised, tender, and inflamed spot on or beneath the skin's surface. Abscesses can develop in various body areas, encompassing the skin, internal organs, and oral cavity.

Bacterial infection is the primary instigator of abscess formation. When bacteria gain access into the body, perhaps via a cut, hair follicle, or obstructed sebaceous gland, the immune system dispatches white blood cells to neutralize the threat. The ensuing immune reaction, combined with deceased bacteria and tissue damage, results in pus buildup within an enclosure, culminating in an abscess.

The dimensions and intensity of abscesses can fluctuate. Minor abscesses might recede spontaneously or with at-home treatments, whereas extensive or deep-rooted abscesses usually necessitate medical intervention. Standard treatment entails the drainage of the abscess to eliminate the pus, and in certain situations, antibiotic administration to eradicate the infection.

Prominent indicators of an abscess encompass localized discomfort, swelling, inflammation, heat, and sensitivity. Occasionally, an abscess may manifest a discernible "head" or pocket filled with pus. If the infection escalates or becomes acute, systemic signs like fever, shivering, and lethargy might arise.

**Home Solutions for Abscesses**:

1. **Warm Compress**: A warm compress can enhance blood flow to the affected zone, fostering recovery and mitigating discomfort.

   - Saturate a clean cloth in tepid water.
   - Extract excess moisture mildly.
   - Position the warm cloth over the abscess for around 10-15 minutes.
   - Redo this a few times daily until the abscess releases its contents and commences healing.

2. **Turmeric Paste**: Turmeric, loaded with antibacterial and anti-inflammatory traits, can be beneficial for abscess treatment.

   - Combine 1 tablespoon of turmeric powder with water to craft a dense paste.

- Smear the concoction directly onto the abscess.

- Shield the region with a sterile cloth or plaster.

- Retain for several hours or overnight.

- Gently cleanse with tepid water.

- Apply this daily until recovery is noticeable.

3. **Garlic Poultice**: Garlic, a natural antimicrobial agent, is effective in addressing abscesses.

- Pulverize some garlic cloves and blend with a dash of olive or coconut oil to form a paste.

- Administer the garlic mixture to the abscess.

- Encase with a sterile cloth or adhesive strip.

- Retain for roughly 30-60 minutes.

- Rinse with lukewarm water.

- Implement this remedy bi-daily until there's an enhancement.

While these remedies can furnish relief, it's pivotal to seek guidance from a medical professional if the abscess aggravates or lacks signs of recuperation. Immediate medical scrutiny for abscesses is crucial, particularly if they're sizable, recurrent, or paired with intense pain or widespread symptoms. Adequate care and oversight are integral to avert further issues and facilitate recovery.

## 2. Acne

Acne is a prevalent dermatological condition manifested as pimples, blackheads, and whiteheads. Effective measures encompass maintaining facial cleanliness, employing non-comedogenic skincare products, refraining from aggressive exfoliation, and exploring topical applications like benzoyl peroxide or salicylic acid.

**Home Remedies for Acne:**

**Tea Tree Oil Spot Treatment:** Blend 1-2 droplets of tea tree oil with 1 teaspoon of coconut oil. Use a cotton bud to dab directly onto acne. Tea tree oil's antibacterial prowess can diminish inflammation and exterminate acne-inducing bacteria.

**Honey and Cinnamon Mask:** Combine 1 tablespoon of honey with 1 teaspoon of cinnamon powder. Spread this concoction on your face, letting it sit for 10-15 minutes before washing off.

Honey's antibacterial attributes paired with cinnamon's anti-inflammatory effects can benefit acne-prone skin.

**Green Tea Toner:** Prepare a green tea infusion and allow it to cool. Utilizing a cotton pad, pat the tea onto your face as a refreshing toner. Green tea's antioxidant components can aid in ameliorating acne and pacifying the skin.

## 3. Aging

Aging denotes the inherent progression of maturing. Although aging is inexorable, upholding a salubrious lifestyle can mitigate some of its repercussions. This entails consuming an antioxidant-abundant diet, maintaining hydration, safeguarding the skin from UV exposure with sunscreen, and consistently exercising.

**Anti-Aging Recipes**:

**Avocado Face Mask**: Pulverize half a mature avocado and amalgamate it with 1 tablespoon of honey. Slather this blend on your face, letting it remain for 15-20 minutes prior to cleansing. Avocado, laden with vitamins and antioxidants, can moisturize and rejuvenate the skin.

**Anti-Aging Smoothie**: Puree 1 cup of spinach, 1/2 cup of berries, half a banana, 1 tablespoon of chia seeds, and 1 cup of almond milk. This beverage brims with antioxidants and vital nutrients that endorse skin health and decelerate the aging trajectory.

**DIY Anti-Aging Serum**: Blend 1 tablespoon of rosehip oil with several droplets of frankincense essential oil. Administer a minuscule quantity of this serum nightly. Rosehip oil, enriched with vitamins A and C, can amplify skin suppleness and attenuate wrinkle visibility.

## 4. Allergies

Allergies transpire when the immune system erroneously responds to typically innocuous entities. Standard mitigative strategies encompass evading allergens, consuming antihistamines, administering nasal mists or eye drops, and consulting healthcare professionals for acute allergic reactions.

**Home Remedies for Allergies**:

**Honey and Lemon Elixir**: Integrate 1 tablespoon of honey with the juice from half a lemon in tepid water. Consume this concoction daily for potential relief from allergic manifestations. Honey can fortify immunity, while lemon possesses innate antihistamine attributes.

**Quercetin-Infused Diet**: Incorporate quercetin-rich produce like apples, onions, broccoli, and citrus fruits into your meals. Quercetin, a natural flavonoid, exhibits anti-allergic characteristics which can temper allergic outbursts.

**Nasal Irrigation**: Leverage a neti pot or saline nasal mist to irrigate your nasal pathways with saline. This aids in expelling allergens and mitigating nasal blockage linked to allergies.

## 5. Asthma

Asthma is a persistent pulmonary ailment marked by episodes of labored breathing, accompanied by wheezing and persistent coughing. Managing this condition often necessitates the use of prescribed inhalers or other medications, steering clear of provocateurs like allergens or external irritants, and upholding a wholesome lifestyle that incorporates consistent physical activity.

**Home Remedies for Asthma**:

**Ginger Tea**: To make this therapeutic brew, immerse freshly sliced ginger in boiling water and steep for 5-10 minutes. Consuming this tea may assist in curtailing inflammation and ameliorating symptoms of asthma.

**Breathing Techniques**: Incorporate deep respiratory exercises into your daily routine to augment pulmonary capacity and oversee asthma manifestations. A beneficial technique is the pursed-lip breathing method: Draw in a breath through your nostrils, counting to two, and then gradually exhale via puckered lips, counting to four.

**Saltwater Gargle**: Combine 1/2 teaspoon of salt with a glass of tepid water. Employ this solution for gargling to assuage a raspy throat or the cough typically associated with asthma.

While these home remedies might offer some relief, it's crucial to remember that asthma can be a severe condition. Always adhere to your doctor's recommendations and prescribed treatments, and seek immediate medical attention if symptoms exacerbate.

## 6. Baby Rash

Babies' tender skin can sometimes develop rashes due to several reasons, including diaper rash, heat rash, or reactions to products. It's essential to keep the skin clean and moisturized, opt for baby-friendly skincare products, make use of special creams for diaper rash, and ensure the baby is not confined in tight clothes or diapers for extended periods.

**Home Remedies for Baby Rash**:

- **Oatmeal Bath**: Immerse your little one in a warm bath infused with fine oatmeal for about 10-15 minutes. Oats possess properties that can calm itchiness and skin irritation.

- **Coconut Oil Application**: Use virgin coconut oil to delicately massage the rash. The moisturizing and anti-inflammatory qualities of coconut oil can provide relief from baby rashes.

- **Chamomile Compress**: Prepare chamomile tea, allow it to cool, immerse a clean cloth in it, and gently apply it to the rash. Chamomile is renowned for its skin-soothing benefits.

## 7. Backache

Back pain can arise from several sources like poor posture, muscle overexertion, or underlying medical conditions. Solutions range from using hot or cold packs, performing mild stretches, taking pain relief medications, ensuring a correct posture, and seeking medical guidance if the pain remains persistent.

**Home Remedies for Backache**:

- **Epsom Salt Soak**: Dissolve 1-2 cups of Epsom salt in a warm bath and immerse yourself for about 20 minutes. Epsom salt can help mitigate muscle tension.

- **Turmeric Milk**: Blend 1 teaspoon of turmeric into a cup of warm milk. Turmeric's anti-inflammatory nature can aid in reducing backache.

- **Gentle Stretches**: Engage in mild stretching to relieve tight muscles. Always consult a medical expert for personalized advice.

## 8. Bites and Strings

The discomfort from insect bites and stings can be mitigated by cleaning the wound, applying a cold press, using topical treatments, ingesting antihistamines, and seeking prompt medical care for severe reactions.

**Home Remedies for Bites and Stings**:

- **Cold Compress**: Alleviate swelling and pain by applying a cloth-covered cold pack to the site.

- **Baking Soda Paste**: Create a mix of baking soda and water and apply to the wound to decrease inflammation and itching.

- **Aloe Vera Application**: Directly apply aloe vera to the site for its soothing benefits.

## 9. Bloating

Bloating results in an uncomfortable fullness in the stomach. To combat this, limit intake of gas-causing foods, consume smaller meals more frequently, try peppermint tea, take OTC gas relief medicines, and remain active.

**Home Remedies for Bloating**:

- **Peppermint Tea**: Sip on peppermint tea post-meals to relax the stomach muscles and diminish bloating.

- **Ginger-Lemon Water**: Add fresh ginger and lemon slices to water and consume the infusion throughout the day to ease bloating.

- **Fennel Seeds**: Post-meals, chew on fennel seeds or prepare fennel seed tea. These seeds can significantly reduce gas and the bloated feeling.

## 10.    Bruise

Bruising happens when blood vessels beneath the skin rupture, leading to a purplish discoloration and tenderness. Immediate application of cold can reduce swelling, while subsequent warmth and gentle massaging can help speed healing.

**Home Remedies for Bruises**:

- **Arnica Salve**: Administer arnica salve or gel to the affected area. Arnica is known for its anti-inflammatory properties which can decrease swelling and discoloration.

- **Cold Compress**: Press a cloth-covered cold compress or ice pack against the bruise for 10-15 minutes to minimize the bruising by constricting blood vessels.

- **Pineapple Consumption**: Drink pineapple juice or place pineapple slices on the bruise. Pineapples have bromelain, which might hasten the bruise's healing.

## 11. Bronchitis

Bronchitis denotes the inflammation of the bronchial tubes, typically resulting from a virus. Recommended remedies involve rest, hydration, using humidifiers, evading irritants like smoke, and taking OTC medicines like cough suppressants.

**Home Remedies for Bronchitis**:

- **Steam Inhalation**: Pour boiling water into a large container. With a towel draped over your head, lean over the container and inhale steam for 10-15 minutes, which can alleviate congestion.

- **Honey Solution**: Combine 1-2 teaspoons of honey in warm water and consume to calm a bronchitis-induced sore throat and cough.

- **Ginger-Garlic Tea**: Steep crushed ginger and garlic in hot water for 10 minutes, strain, and drink. These ingredients have antimicrobial and anti-inflammatory properties beneficial for respiratory issues.

## 12. Burns and Sunburns

Immediate cooling with cold water can mitigate pain from minor burns. For treatment, apply aloe vera gel, antibiotic ointments, and cover with a sterile dressing. Sunburns can be addressed similarly, complemented by soothing lotions and pain relievers if needed.

**Home Remedies for Burns**:

- **Aloe Vera Application**: Directly apply aloe vera gel on burns. Known for its cooling and moisturizing abilities, it can hasten skin recovery.

- **Milk Compress**: Drench a cloth in cold milk and place it on the burn. The milk's coolness and proteins can reduce inflammation and pain.

- **Apple Cider Vinegar Mix**: Blend apple cider vinegar with water in equal ratios. Using a cotton ball, dab the solution on the burn, providing pain relief and minimizing the risk of infections.

## 13.    Canker Sore

Canker sores are painful mouth ulcers. Alleviate them by steering clear of spicy or acidic foods, employing OTC treatments, and practicing good oral hygiene.

**Home Remedies for Canker Sores**:

- **Saltwater Gargle**: In warm water, dissolve a teaspoon of salt. Use the solution as a mouth rinse for 30 seconds before spitting. This rinse can decrease inflammation and accelerate healing.

- **Turmeric-Honey Paste**: Combine honey with a bit of turmeric to form a paste. Place it on the sore. While honey fights bacteria, turmeric, with its anti-inflammatory attributes, can reduce sore pain.

- **Coconut Oil Swishing**: Hold coconut oil in your mouth and swish for 10-15 minutes, then spit. This method can help decrease inflammation and promote sore healing.

## 14.    Cold Sores

These are fluid-filled blisters around the lips caused by the herpes simplex virus. Using antiviral treatments and avoiding direct contact can prevent its spread.

**Home Remedies for Cold Sores:**

- **Lemon Balm Treatment:** Directly rub lemon balm salve on the cold sore. It can help shorten and lessen the sore due to its antiviral nature.

- **Cooling Compress:** Use a cloth-encased ice pack on the cold sore for 10-15 minutes to relieve pain and diminish swelling.

- **Lysine Intake:** Consume lysine supplements as guided by a medical professional. Lysine might counteract the herpes virus.

## 15.    Constipation

To address constipation, it's recommended to drink ample water, eat foods abundant in fiber such as whole grains, fruits, and veggies, maintain regular physical activity, and, if needed, resort to non-prescription laxatives or stool enhancers. Cultivating consistent bowel routines and pinpointing the root reasons for constipation are vital.

## Home Remedies for Constipation:

- **High-Fiber Drink:** Combine 1 cup each of spinach and almond milk, a mature banana, and a tablespoon of chia seeds. Rich in fiber, this blended beverage can encourage regularity.

- **Morning or Night Prune Drink:** Sip on a glass of prune juice either at the start of your day or before retiring to bed. Prunes, being natural bowel stimulants, can assist in mitigating constipation.

- **Flax Drink:** Stir in a tablespoon of crushed flaxseeds into a glass of water and let it rest for an hour or two. Consume this to enhance stool volume and alleviate constipation.

## 16.    Couch and Cold

When faced with cough and cold indications, suggested treatments encompass sufficient rest, adequate hydration, over-the-counter remedies like cough inhibitors, lozenges for the throat, and decongestants for the nose. Employing steam breathing techniques and saltwater nasal sprays are also beneficial.

## Home Remedies for Couch and Cold:

- **Ginger-Honey Infusion:** Make a ginger tea and blend in 1-2 spoons of honey. The ginger helps with inflammation, whereas honey provides relief for throat irritation and curtails cough. Essential Oil

- **Steam Breathing:** Into a container of boiling water, introduce several droplets of either eucalyptus or peppermint essential oils. Encase your head with a cloth, shield your eyes, and breathe in the steam for about 10-15 minutes. This method aids in clearing blocked nasal passages and soothing cough-related discomfort.

- **Nourishing Chicken Broth:** Craft a traditional chicken broth, incorporating veggies, garlic, and aromatic herbs. The soup's heat and vapor are comforting during coughs and colds, and its components can bolster immunity.

## 17. Diarrhea

During bouts of diarrhea, maintaining hydration with electrolyte-enriched fluids is essential. Opting for mild foods such as rice, bread, and bananas can calm the stomach. While drugs like loperamide can offer immediate relief, addressing the root issue and seeking medical advice if the condition continues is vital.

**Home Remedies for Diarrhea:**

**Hydration and Electrolyte Solutions:**

**Recipe:** Create a DIY hydration solution with 1 liter of water, a pinch of salt (1 teaspoon), and 4 spoons of sugar. You might also add natural juices like apple or cranberry, or opt for coconut water and herbal infusions.

**Solution:** Consume clear and electrolyte-abundant beverages to replenish fluids and minerals lost from diarrhea. These liquids combat dehydration and offer necessary nourishment.

**BRAT Regimen:**

**Recipe:** The BRAT regimen focuses on simple, low-fiber consumables: bananas, rice, apple puree, and bread. Whip up some plain rice paired with boiled and mashed bananas. Also, consider plain bread toast and unsweetened apple mash.

**Solution:** This diet is mild on the digestive system, aiding in stool solidification during episodes of diarrhea. The ingredients provide readily absorbed carbs and can mitigate diarrhea's effects.

**Ginger Infusion:**

**Recipe:** Shred some raw ginger and immerse it in hot water for a duration of 10-15 minutes. After filtering, sweeten with honey as per preference.

**Solution:** Ginger is renowned for its anti-inflammatory and germ-fighting attributes, potentially easing the gut and diminishing diarrhea-related discomfort. A cup of this tea can be soothing..

## 18. Dry Skin

To address dry skin, consistent moisturization using unscented lotions, avoiding scalding water during baths or showers, opting for mild skin cleansers, and shielding the skin from extreme climatic conditions with suitable attire are recommended. Utilizing humidifiers can also elevate indoor moisture levels.

**Home Remedies for Dry Skin:**

- **Oat-infused Bath:** Incorporate either colloidal oatmeal or ground oats into a tepid bath, immersing yourself for about 15-20 minutes. Oats are renowned for their ability to ease skin dryness and discomfort.

- **Natural Coconut Moisturizer:** Smear pure coconut oil on parched skin patches. Recognized for its hydrating qualities, coconut oil deeply moisturizes and rejuvenates the skin.

- **Nourishing Facial Mask:** Combine a mashed half avocado with a spoon of honey and a spoon of unflavored yogurt. Apply this blend on the face, allowing it to sit for roughly 15-20 minutes before washing off. The trio - avocado, honey, and yogurt - are potent moisturizers, ideal for reviving dehydrated skin.

## 19. Earache

Various reasons can lead to earaches, ranging from infections within the ear to accumulated earwax. Relief might be found by placing a warm pack over the painful ear, opting for over-the-counter analgesics, or employing ear drops designed for wax elimination. However, seeking advice from a medical expert becomes imperative if the discomfort is persistent or intensifies.

**Home Remedies for Earache:**

- **Heated Relief:** Place a warm cloth or heating pad on the aching ear for a duration of 10-15 minutes. The applied warmth can aid in decreasing pain and curbing inflammation.

- **Garlic-Infused Oil:** Crush a piece of garlic and merge it with lukewarm olive oil. Allow the concoction to sit briefly for about 10 minutes and then filter the oil. With a sanitized dropper, introduce a few drops of the oil concoction into the problematic ear. Owing to its antimicrobial attributes, garlic can be beneficial in mitigating ear discomfort.

- **Common Pain Alleviators:** Consider taking non-prescription pain alleviators like acetaminophen or ibuprofen, adhering strictly to the prescribed dose. They can offer temporary relief from ear pain.

## 20. Eczema

Eczema results in dry, inflamed, and often itchy skin patches. Relief may come from frequent moisturizing using hypoallergenic lotions, circumventing irritants, preferring tepid showers or baths, applying doctor-prescribed creams or ointments, and monitoring stress.

**Home Remedies for Eczema:**

- **Soothing Oatmeal Soak:** Add either colloidal oatmeal or well-grounded oats to a bath and immerse for about 15-20 minutes. Oats have the capacity to mitigate the itch and redness linked to eczema.
- **Natural Coconut Balm:** Directly spread virgin coconut oil over the impacted skin regions. This oil serves as an innate hydrator, potentially alleviating eczema's dryness and discomfort.
- **Evening Primrose Supplement:** As advised by a medical expert, consume evening primrose oil supplements. It's rich in gamma-linolenic acid, known to counteract inflammation and possibly ease eczema signs.

## 21. Fatigue

Multiple factors, like insufficient sleep, stress, or medical conditions, can cause fatigue. Solutions are ample rest, a wholesome diet, consistent physical activity, effective stress management, and tending to any health issues.

**Home Remedies for Fatigue:**

- **Vitality Booster Smoothie:** Whisk a banana, some spinach, 1 tablespoon of almond paste, almond milk (1 cup), with a pinch of cinnamon. This nutritious mix may elevate vitality.
- **Peppermint Aromatherapy:** Inhale peppermint essential oil straight or using a vaporizer. Its refreshing properties can potentially dissipate fatigue and sharpen concentration.
- **Routine Movement:** Maintain consistent activity, perhaps light jogging, brisk strolls, or yoga. Such activities can amplify energy and combat weariness.

## 22.    Fever

Fever usually signals an ongoing bodily combat against infections. Resolutions encompass ample fluid intake, relaxation, donning breathable outfits, administering non-prescription fever-lowering drugs (following guidelines), and if persistent or intense, medical consultation.

**Home Remedies for Fever:**

- **Fluid Boost:** Consume adequate liquids, like water, teas, or clear broths, aiding hydration and fever support.
- **Cooling Cloth:** Use a cloth drenched in cool water on the forehead or other hotspots to possibly lessen body heat.
- **Repose:** Secure abundant rest, facilitating recuperation.

## 23.    Flatulence

To alleviate flatulence, one may sidestep foods like legumes or sodas that induce gas, consume at a measured pace, consider over-the-counter drugs with simethicone, and ensure consistent motion.

**Home Remedies for Flatulence:**

- **Gas-easing Peppermint Brew:** After meals, sip on a freshly prepared peppermint tea. Peppermint's natural properties can curtail gas.
- **Ginger Drink:** Allow fresh ginger slices to steep in boiling water for a quarter hour. Sip this ginger liquid to counter gas.
- **Fennel Elixir:** Submerge a spoon of fennel seeds in boiling water for 10 minutes, strain and drink. This can offset gas and bloating.

## 24.    Flu

For flu manifestations, consider ample rest, hydration, over-the-counter pain and fever medications, warm salt gargles for throat soreness, and if symptoms exacerbate or linger, medical attention.

**Home Remedies for Flu:**

- **Lemon-Honey Hot Beverage:** Combine lemon juice (from half a lemon) and honey (1-2 teaspoons) in heated water. Consuming this can alleviate flu discomforts.

- **Antimicrobial Garlic Broth:** Craft a broth using garlic, chosen veggies, and either chicken or veggie stock. Garlic bolsters immunity during flu bouts.
- **Recuperation Support:** Rest and hydration are vital. Ingest plenty of liquids, from herbal infusions to clear broths, ensuring hydration and immunity boost.

## 25. Gingivities

Gingivitis refers to gum inflammation, commonly resulting from inadequate oral care. Effective solutions involve brushing teeth diligently twice daily, daily flossing, using antimicrobial mouth rinses, and consistent dental appointments.

**Home Remedies for Gingivities:**

- **Salt Rinse**: Mix 1/2 teaspoon of salt in warm water. Gargle for 30 seconds and spit out. This can help lower inflammation and battle harmful oral bacteria.

- **Tea Tree Rinse**: Combine 2-3 drops of tea tree oil in warm water. Gargle and spit after 30 seconds. Tea tree oil's antimicrobial properties can help treat gingivitis.

- **Routine Oral Care**: Ensure you brush twice daily, floss every day, and utilize an antibacterial mouth rinse. Good oral care is crucial to prevent and treat gingivitis.

## 26. Hair Loss

Various factors, including genetics, hormonal fluctuations, or medical conditions, can lead to hair loss. Possible remedies include a nutritious diet, avoiding aggressive hair treatments, gentle hair products, managing stress, and consulting a doctor for persistent hair thinning.

**Home Remedies for Hair Loss:**

- **Essential Oil Massage**: Blend rosemary or lavender oil with a carrier oil like coconut. Massage on your scalp, leaving it for several hours before washing.

- **Nutritious Diet**: Consume nutrient-rich foods beneficial for hair, like lean protein, fish, eggs, nuts, greens, and fruits.

- **Kind Hair Care**: Steer clear of harmful treatments, avoid high heat styling, and refrain from pulling hair into tight styles. Choose gentle shampoos and don't rub hair aggressively after washing.

## 27.  Halitosis

Halitosis, or bad breath, emits an off-putting scent from the mouth. Regular oral care, tongue cleaning, and antimicrobial mouth rinses can treat it. Sugar-free gum or mints can offer temporary freshness. Drink ample water and avoid odor-causing foods like garlic for improved breath.

**Home Remedies for Halitosis:**

- **Oil Pulling**: Swish coconut oil in your mouth for 10-15 minutes, then spit. This can help diminish bacteria and enhance oral health.

- **Herbal Rinse**: Make an herbal tea using ingredients like peppermint. After cooling and straining, use it as a mouthwash post-brushing.

- **Tongue Cleaning**: Regularly clean your tongue to remove bacteria, helping to minimize bad breath

## 28.  Hangover

A hangover follows excessive alcohol intake, presenting with fatigue, headache, nausea, and dehydration. Remedies encompass hydration, electrolyte replenishment, and nutrient-rich meals. Herbal teas can provide stomach relief. Rest and avoiding alcohol speed up recovery.

**Home Remedies for Hangover:**

- **Hydration**: Drink water or hydration solutions to counter dehydration from alcohol. Regularly sip water during the day.

- **Electrolyte Foods**: Eat electrolyte-dense foods like bananas or coconut water.

- **Detox Water**: Use ginger and lemon slices in water. After infusion, drink the mixture to help digestion.

## 29.  Headache

Headaches can arise from various sources, including tension, sinus issues, dehydration, or migraines. Potential remedies include resting in dim, silent areas, applying temperature compresses, relaxation techniques, and OTC pain medications. Identifying triggers is key.

**Home Remedies for Headache:**

- **Peppermint Treatment**: Mix peppermint oil with a carrier oil. Apply and massage on pain areas for relief.

- **Cool Compress**: Place a chilled cloth or ice pack on your forehead or neck for relief.

- **Hydration**: Drinking water can prevent dehydration-induced headaches.

## 30. Reflux

Reflux or GERD occurs when stomach acid enters the esophagus, causing heartburn and discomfort. Remedies involve avoiding certain foods, consuming smaller meals, staying upright post-meals, and not sleeping immediately after eating. OTC treatments can offer relief, but chronic symptoms require medical consultation.

**Home Remedies for Reflux:**

- **Vinegar Solution**: Mix raw apple cider vinegar in warm water and drink before meals for relief.

- **Slippery Elm Drink**: Drink slippery elm tea post-meals for a soothing effect.

- **Sleeping Posture**: Elevate your bed's head or use a wedge pillow to prevent nighttime reflux.

## 31. Stress

Stress affects both mental and physical health. To manage stress, incorporate relaxation techniques, regular exercise, balanced diets, sufficient sleep, and engaging in enjoyable activities. Professional therapy can also be beneficial.

**Home Remedies for Stress:**

- **Deep Breathing**: Engage in deep breathing exercises for relaxation.
- **Mindfulness**: Dedicate time for daily meditation or mindfulness practices.
- **Calming Teas**: Consume teas like chamomile or lavender to aid relaxation.

# Chapter 2: Herbs to Use in the Kitchen

Herbs play a dual role in our lives; they serve both medicinal and culinary purposes. By integrating herbs into daily meals, one can elevate taste profiles while simultaneously reaping various health rewards. Explore how these plants can bring a blend of flavor and wellness to your table.

- **Basil**

  - **Description:** A fragrant herb, basil has bright green leaves and offers a mix of sweetness with a hint of pepper.

  - **Cooking Applications:** Essential in Mediterranean dishes, basil is found in pastas, pestos, salads, and various soups.

  - **Health Aspects:** Rich in vitamins A and K, antioxidants, and having antibacterial capabilities, basil can boost immunity, soothe inflammation, and aid digestion.

- **Rosemary**

  - **Description:** An evergreen plant, rosemary has sharp leaves and emits a strong, pine-scented aroma.

  - **Cooking Applications:** It's a choice herb for roast meats, vegetables, bread, and flavoring marinades.

  - **Health Aspects:** A source of antioxidants, rosemary can bolster respiratory health, digestion, and might even sharpen memory.

- **Thyme**

  - **Description:** A tiny perennial, thyme boasts small aromatic leaves with a gentle, earthy taste.

  - **Cooking Applications:** Used in dishes ranging from stews to roasted meats, thyme is cherished in Mediterranean and French meals.

  - **Health Aspects:** With essential oils boasting antibacterial effects, thyme can assist with digestion and respiratory support.

- **Oregano**

  - **Description:** Oregano's bold scent and somewhat bitter palate make it a recognized culinary herb.

  - **Cooking Applications:** Fundamental in Greek and Italian cuisines, it spices up pizzas, sauces, and dressings.

- **Health Aspects:** Oregano, being antioxidant-rich and antimicrobial, can boost the immune system and aid digestive processes.

- **Parsley**

  - **Description:** Parsley, a biennial herb, is vibrant green with a crisp, slightly peppery taste.

  - **Cooking Applications:** Beyond garnishing, parsley enriches salads, soups, and marinades.

  - **Health Aspects:** Packed with vitamins A, C, and K, parsley aids in bone health, digestion, and has diuretic attributes.

- **Dill**

  - **Description:** A unique herb, dill has soft leaves with a taste that merges licorice and citrus.

  - **Cooking Applications:** Ideal for pickles, seafood, and dressings, dill brings a fresh element to recipes.

  - **Health Aspects:** Its essential oils offer antimicrobial effects, aiding digestion and providing a calming sensation.

- **Mint**

  - **Description:** A perennial plant, mint has aromatic leaves with a cooling, sweet flavor.

  - **Cooking Applications:** Versatile in sweet and savory meals, it's used in teas, desserts, and even mixed drinks.

  - **Health Aspects:** Mint can alleviate nausea, aid digestion, and refresh the breath.

When you incorporate herbs into your dishes, you're offering a blend of flavor and health to those you serve. From basil's aromatic charm to thyme's grounding essence, each herb holds its own unique presence. Experiment with their pairings and let creativity lead the way. For optimal flavor and nutrition, always opt for fresh herbs.

Consider setting up your own herb garden, ensuring you always have these culinary gems at your fingertips. Whether in a small pot by a window or a full-fledged garden, cultivating herbs can be a rewarding venture.

Utilizing these herbs not only elevates the taste of meals but potentially offers health boons. These plants can boost one's health organically, from immune enhancement to aiding digestion.

Embrace these herbs, letting them guide you on a culinary exploration that tantalizes the taste buds while nourishing the body and soul. Let their vibrant flavors and healing attributes infuse your meals, turning every dish into a fulfilling experience.

Delve into the world of culinary herbs and let the adventure begin!

Note: While culinary use of these herbs is generally safe, it's advisable not to consume them medicinally without consulting with a healthcare professional or knowledgeable herbalist.

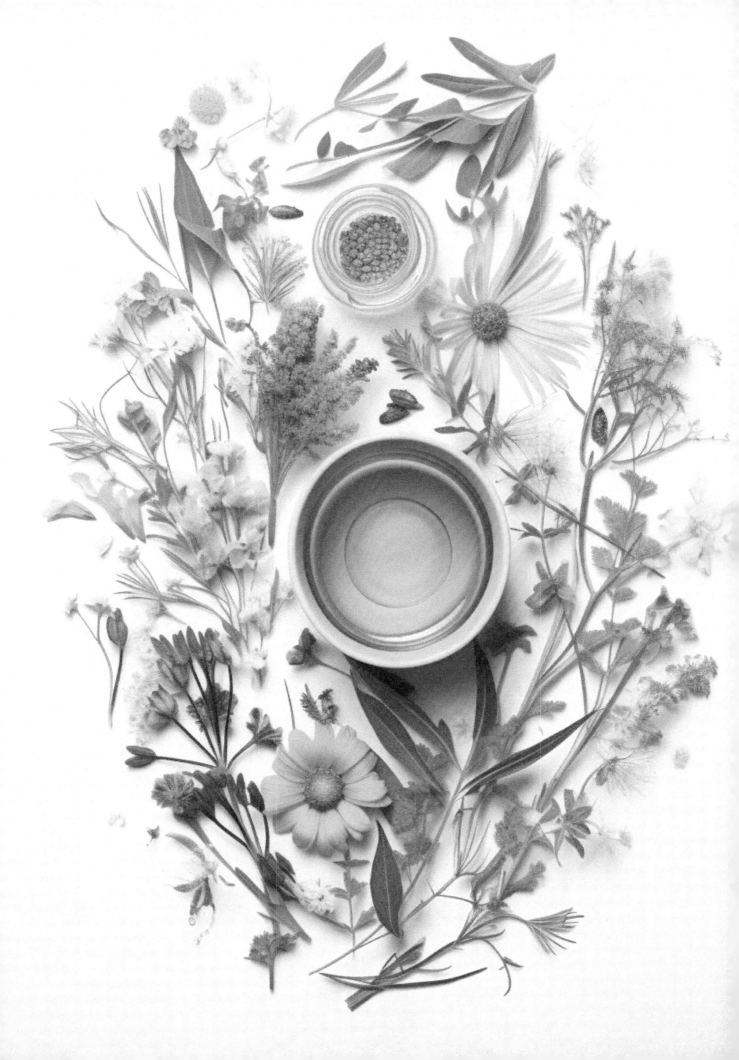

# BOOK 7: HEALING INFUSIONS AND HERBAL TEA

## Introduction

Welcome to the serene world of healing infusions and herbal tea, where nature's tranquility meets age-old medicinal wisdom. This guide aims to journey with readers through the myriad benefits of herbal teas and their storied past. Venture with us into the depths of herb lore, uncovering their profound secrets and guiding you towards a path of complete wellness. Our blends span from gentle floral concoctions to robust, invigorating brews.

In today's fast-paced society, there's a burgeoning desire to reconnect with the Earth and seek solace in her nurturing embrace. Herbal teas serve as a bridge to this harmonious bond, reminding us to pause, savor the moment, and internally rejuvenate. Historically, across global civilizations, people have tapped into the healing prowess of plants, leveraging their gifts to enhance physical vitality, restore balance, and uplift the spirit.

Throughout this volume, we pay tribute to the timeless art of herbal healing, celebrating its ability to comfort, heal, and rejuvenate. Embark on an adventure with us, immersing in the captivating scents, vibrant hues, and distinct flavors that each herb blend presents. Every herb, from the gentle chamomile blossoms to the invigorating ginger roots, holds a unique tale and allure.

Beyond discussing individual ingredients, this book delves into the artistry of blending and the magic of infusion. Understand the techniques that transform a simple tea experience into a moment of wonder. Master the art of balancing flavors, enhancing aromas, and creating custom blends that cater to your unique needs. Whether you seek relaxation, vigor, or introspection, there's an ideal herbal infusion awaiting your discovery.

Herbal teas' advantages extend far beyond their sensory delights. They offer tangible health benefits, enhancing our physical and mental states. From aiding digestion and bolstering immunity to promoting restful sleep and reducing anxiety, the healing potential of these teas is vast and varied. Together, we'll delve into the therapeutic attributes of numerous herbs, understanding their role in fostering health and balance.

By the book's conclusion, you'll be armed with knowledge and inspiration. We offer a comprehensive guide on sourcing, harvesting, and preserving herbs to retain their utmost purity and potency. Learn to craft, blend, and tailor your brews aligning with your health aspirations. From brewing techniques to blending protocols, we've got you covered.

So, ready your favorite teacup, inhale deeply, and join us on this expedition into the therapeutic realm of herbal teas. Allow the warmth of the brew and the nuanced herbal interplay to transport you to a place of serenity. With this book as your trusted guide, embark on a transformative journey, connecting deeply with nature and nourishing your body, mind, and soul in the process.

# Chapter 1: Herbal Therapy in the Modern Age

In our contemporary world, there's a growing gravitation towards natural and holistic health solutions, with herbal therapy standing out as a prime choice. By marrying age-old wisdom and practices with today's scientific innovations, herbal therapy has become a prominent fixture in modern health and wellness discussions. We'll venture into the essence of herbal therapy, examining its revival, its scientific foundations, and its significance in fostering a balanced and healthful existence.

## Rediscovering Herbal Medicine

Herbal medicine's renaissance speaks to a transformation in our healthcare inclinations. Recent times have witnessed a burgeoning curiosity in nature's remedies, spurred on by varying reasons – from critiques of mainstream medicine and yearnings for personalized healthcare to deeper bonds with the environment. We'll probe into this revival, understanding the growing calls for greener and more universally accessible health avenues.

## Scientific Foundations of Herbal Medicine

Far from being mere tales and traditions, herbal therapy has strong roots in science. We'll journey through the rigorous research that underscores the potency of herbal solutions and their intrinsic components. This deep dive will illuminate the medicinal attributes of various plants – their ability to combat microbes, reduce inflammation, and neutralize free radicals. A comprehension of this scientific facet enhances our appreciation of herbal remedies as valid complements to standard treatments.

## Integrating Tradition and Innovation

Crucial to holistic healing is the melding of time-honored herbal insights with contemporary health paradigms. We'll dissect how herbal treatments can be harmoniously intertwined with standard medical practices, presenting a well-rounded, individualized health approach. By valuing age-old knowledge and the latest in scientific breakthroughs, we're navigating a route towards a health system that offers the pinnacle of both epochs.

## The Role of Herbalists and Practitioners

The linchpins of herbal therapy are the herbalists and specialists, steering individuals towards peak health. We'll demystify the expertise, ethical stances, and roles of these professionals, emphasizing their pivotal contributions in offering bespoke health roadmaps and unwavering support. The synergy between herbalists and traditional health providers is key in architecting a unified, patient-centric health strategy.

## Integrating Herbal Remedies Daily

Herbal therapy unveils myriad ways to weave nature's cures into our quotidian routines. We'll delve into pragmatic methods of employing herbal concoctions, from brewing teas to relying on tinctures and supplements. By understanding the vast applications of common herbs, we can harness their multifaceted health benefits – be it bolstering immunity, fostering restful sleep, or simply managing daily stress.

## Safety and Regulation in Herbal Therapy

Like all healthcare avenues, prioritizing safety and maintaining standards is crucial. We'll delve into the oversight and quality benchmarks for herbal goods, emphasizing the importance of ethical sourcing, production, and product marking. By equipping individuals with insights about the safety and rules associated with herbal items, we can foster knowledgeable choices and encourage their judicious use. Herbal therapy, with its reemergence and blending of age-old practices with modern science, provides a comprehensive way to wellness. Grasping the scientific foundations of herbal treatments, the contributions of its professionals, and ways to weave them into our daily lives enables us to utilize nature's therapeutic prowess to foster health and harmony. As we further navigate the herbal therapy landscape, appreciating the profound impact of botanicals and their role in our inherent healing mechanisms is vital.

The revival of herbal remedies highlights a paradigm shift in our health perspectives and an inclination towards greener, more accessible healthcare solutions. The allure of nature's innate knowledge is drawing more individuals, leading them to solutions that resonate with their beliefs and connect them more profoundly with the environment. Herbal therapy, in its essence, not only presents a plethora of treatments but also promotes a mindful, all-encompassing approach to personal wellness.

Scientific endeavors have been instrumental in affirming the potency of herbal treatments. Through meticulous research and technological strides, we've deepened our grasp on the primary constituents in medicinal flora and their specific healing attributes. This information creates a bridge between age-old botanical practices and current scientific knowledge, paving the way for data-driven herbal remedies.

The fusion of time-honored practices and modern innovations is pivotal to fully realizing herbal therapy's potential. Respecting the teachings handed down over eras and integrating modern research and tools, we can outline a holistic and potent therapeutic strategy. Teamwork among herbal professionals, regular healthcare specialists, and doctors is essential for presenting patients with a comprehensive, tailor-made health blueprint catering to individual requisites.

Herbal treatments aren't just solutions to particular health issues; they are versatile tools for overall wellness enhancement. Whether it's sipping a calming herbal brew, integrating plant-based concentrates in daily habits, or concocting health-boosting herbal blends, these habits encourage a renewed bond with the natural realm and a deeper introspection.

Upholding stringent rules and ensuring quality is vital in the domain of herbal treatments. Ethical procurement, standardized production, and transparent product indications vouch for the genuineness and reliability of herbal items. It's imperative for users to stay abreast of the nuances of herbal item safety and guidelines, allowing them to make informed choices and opt for trusted products from credible vendors.

Embracing botanical remedies connects us to nature's restorative essence, fortifying our physical, mental, and emotional faculties in our quest for peak health. Be it through therapeutic brews or herbal concoctions, herbal therapy beckons us to unearth the time-tested insights encapsulated in the botanical realm, setting us on a trajectory of comprehensive rejuvenation and enlightenment.

# Chapter 2: Recipes

Herbal therapy, sometimes referred to as phytotherapy or herbal medicine, entails employing plant-based materials and their derivatives for healing purposes. Though it's crucial to seek advice from a medical expert before venturing into any herbal treatments, I can offer a basic overview of herbal practices and a couple of formulas using widespread herbs. Bear in mind, it's essential to proceed with care, since people can respond differently to specific herbs, and certain herbs might interfere with prescribed drugs or may not be suitable for some medical situations.

## 1. Relaxation Chamomile Tea:

**Ingredients:**

- 1 tbsp dried chamomile petals
- 1 cup hot water
- Optional: honey or lemon for flavoring

**Instructions:**

- Put chamomile in a teapot or infuser.
- Add the hot water to the chamomile.
- Steep for 5-10 mins.
- Filter and mix in honey or lemon as preferred.
- Drink it for relaxation or before sleep.

Chamomile's calming effects assist in easing stress and enhancing sleep.

## 2. Ginger-Turmeric Health Shot:

**Ingredients:**

- 1-inch fresh ginger, skinned
- 1-inch fresh turmeric, skinned
- 1 lemon's juice
- Touch of black pepper (boosts turmeric uptake)
- Optional: small amount of cayenne peppe

**Instructions:**

- Juice or blend ginger and turmeric.
- Incorporate lemon juice and black pepper.
- Optionally, mix in cayenne pepper for added zing.
- Stir and take as a concentrated shot.
- Refrigerate any excess up to 3 days.

This robust shot, when taken daily, helps in maintaining wellness and decreasing bodily inflammation.

## 3. Skin Relief Calendula Ointment:

**Ingredients:**

- 1 cup calendula petals (either dried or fresh)
- 1 cup base oil (like olive or sweet almond oil)
- 1 oz. beeswax (shredded or in pellet form)
- Optional: 10 drops lavender essential oil for fragrance

**Instructions:**

- Combine calendula petals and the chosen oil in a jar that's heat-resistant.
- Set the jar in a pot filled with water to form a double boiler.
- Slowly heat for 2-3 hours, stirring occasionally.
- Filter the oil and discard petals.
- Reheat the oil with beeswax until it fully melts.
- Take off the heat and optionally mix in lavender oil.
- Decant into small jars and let it cool.

Apply the calendula ointment to minor skin wounds, burns, or parched skin to aid healing.

## 4. Echinacea Immune-Boosting Tincture:

**Ingredients:**

- 1 cup echinacea (dried)
- 2 cups vodka or another high-proof spirit

**Instructions:**

- Add dried echinacea to a jar.
- Cover with vodka or spirit.
- Close the jar and give it a good shake.
- Store in a shaded cool area for 4-6 weeks, shaking intermittently.
- Once ready, filter the liquid.
- Store in dropper bottles for dosage control.
- For immune support, take 1-2 dropper amounts daily during flu season.

Echinacea is famed for its ability to enhance immunity, often utilized to lessen cold and flu intensity.

## 5. Digestive Peppermint-Ginger Tea:

**Ingredients:**

- 1 tbsp dried peppermint
- 1 tbsp dried ginger
- 2 cups hot water
- Optional: honey or lemon for flavor

**Instructions:**

- Add peppermint and ginger to a teapot or infuser.
- Pour hot water over the herbs.
- Steep for 10-15 mins.
- Filter and mix in honey or lemon if you like.
- Consume post meals to aid digestion.

Both peppermint and ginger are celebrated for their digestive properties.

## 6. Lavender Sleep Pillow:

**Ingredients:**

- 1 cup dried lavender
- 1 cup dried chamomile
- 1 cup dried rose petals
- Materials for sachet creation: cloth, needle, and thread

**Instructions:**

- Combine the three dried herbs in a bowl.
- Cut two cloth pieces in your chosen shape.
- With the outer sides in, sew three edges.
- Stuff the sachet with the mixed herbs.
- Sew shut the final edge.
- Position beneath your pillow for better sleep.

This sleep sachet amalgamates chamomile, rose, and lavender for peaceful rest.

## 7. Stress-Relief Lavender Bath Salts:

**Ingredients:**

- 1 cup Epsom salts
- 1/2 cup sea salts
- 1/4 cup dried lavender
- 10-15 drops lavender essential oil

**Instructions:**

- In a mixing bowl, combine the salts and dried lavender.
- Add the essential oil and mix well.
- Store in a sealed jar.
- Use 1/2-1 cup in a warm bath and soak for 20-30 mins.

This bath salt mix is designed to alleviate tension and relax the body.

## 8. Anxiety-Relief Lemon Balm Tincture:

**Ingredients:**

- 1 cup fresh lemon balm leaves

- 2 cups vodka or another strong spirit

**Instructions:**

- Clean and dry the lemon balm leaves.
- Cut them into small pieces and place in a jar.
- Pour over vodka or spirit.
- Seal the jar and shake.
- Keep in a dark, cool space for 4-6 weeks, occasionally shaking.
- Once done, strain and bottle.
- To ease anxiety, take 1-2 dropper amounts as needed.

Lemon balm is esteemed for its ability to uplift and soothe the mind.

## 9. Arnica Salve for Muscle Pain:

**Ingredients:**

- 1/2 cup dried arnica flowers
- 1 cup base oil (like coconut or olive)
- 1 oz. beeswax (in pellet form or shredded)

**Instructions:**

- Combine the arnica flowers and oil in a heat-proof jar.
- Prepare a water bath by placing the jar in a pot filled with water.
- Warm gently for 2-3 hours.
- Strain out the arnica from the oil.
- In a clean container, warm the infused oil and melt in the beeswax.
- Pour into containers and allow to cool and solidify.

Use this salve on sore muscles to provide relief. Note: Do not apply to broken skin or open wounds.

## 10. Soothing Lavender Infusion:

**Ingredients:**

- 1 tbsp. lavender buds, dried
- 1 cup water, hot
- Optional: honey or lemon for flavoring

**Instructions:**

- Add dried lavender to a teapot or tea strainer.
- Introduce the hot water to the lavender.
- Allow it to sit for 5-10 minutes.
- Sieve the drink and mix in honey or lemon if you prefer.
- Drink the lavender blend to unwind and relieve stress.

## 11. Elderberry Immunity Tea:

**Ingredients:**

- 2 tbsp. elderberries, dried
- 1 tsp. echinacea, dried
- 1 tsp. rose hips, dried
- 2 cups water, hot
- Optional: honey or lemon for flavoring

**Instructions:**

- In a teapot or strainer, mix elderberries, echinacea, and rose hips.
- Introduce the hot water to the mixed herbs.
- Let it sit for 15-20 minutes.
- Sieve the tea and enhance with honey or lemon if you like.
- Consume this tea frequently for immunity benefits.

## 12. Digestive Calendula Tea:

**Ingredients:**

- 1 tbsp. calendula buds, dried
- 1 tbsp. peppermint, dried
- 2 cups water, hot
- Optional: honey or lemon for flavoring

**Instructions:**

- Add calendula and peppermint to a teapot or tea strainer.
- Introduce the hot water to the herbs.
- Allow to infuse for 10-15 minutes.
- Sieve the tea, and mix in honey or lemon if preferred.
- Sip this blend post meals to support digestion.

## 13. Refreshing Mint Lemonade:

**Ingredients:**

- 2 tbsp. peppermint leaves, dried
- 4 cups water, cold
- Juice from 2 lemons
- Optional: honey or sugar for sweetness

**Instructions:**

- Combine peppermint and water in a jug.
- Let it infuse in the fridge for 4 hours or overnight.
- Filter the liquid, discarding peppermint.
- Incorporate lemon juice and sweeten as per taste.
- Serve chilled for a revitalizing experience.

## 14. Nourishing Nettle Infusion:

**Ingredients:**

- 2 tbsp. nettle, dried
- 2 cups water, hot

**Instructions:**

- Introduce dried nettle to a teapot or strainer.
- Pour hot water over the nettle.
- Allow it to infuse for 15-20 minutes.
- Filter the drink and get rid of nettle leaves.
- Savor this nutritious infusion for its mineral richness.

## 15. Soothing Lemon Balm Beverage:

**Ingredients:**

- 1 tbsp. lemon balm, dried
- 1 cup water, hot
- Optional: honey or lemon for flavoring

**Instructions:**

- Add dried lemon balm to a teapot or tea strainer.

- Pour the hot water over it.
- Let it infuse for 5-10 minutes.
- Strain and flavor with honey or lemon if desired.
- Consume this serene blend for relaxation and anxiety relief.

## 16. Rosemary Concentration Tea:

**Ingredients:**

- 1 tbsp. dried rosemary
- 1 cup hot water
- Optional: honey or lemon

**Instructions:**

- Introduce dried rosemary to a teapot or infuser.
- Add the boiling water.
- Allow to sit for 5-10 mins.
- Sieve, and add flavor enhancers if preferred.
- Sip this for heightened focus and cognitive sharpness.

## 17. Nightly Valerian Brew:

**Ingredients:**

- 1 tbsp. valerian root, dried
- 1 cup hot water
- Optional: honey

**Instructions:**

- Add valerian root to a teapot or infuser.
- Introduce the boiling water.
- Infuse for 10-15 mins.
- Filter, and sweeten if liked.
- Consume before sleep for tranquility.

## 18. Energizing Ginseng Infusion:

**Ingredients:**

- 1 tsp. ginseng root, dried
- 1 cup hot water
- Optional: honey or lemon

**Instructions:**

- Introduce dried ginseng to a teapot or infuser.
- Add boiling water.
- Let sit for 5-10 mins.
- Strain and optionally flavor.
- Drink for a vitality uplift.

## 19. Refreshing Lemongrass Iced Tea:

**Ingredients:**

- 2 tbsp. dried lemongrass
- 4 cups hot water
- Optional: honey, sugar, and mint leaves for garnishing

**Instructions:**

- Add lemongrass to a pitcher.
- Introduce boiling water.
- Infuse for 10-15 mins.
- Sieve, sweeten if needed, and refrigerate.
- Serve chilled, with mint if preferred.

## 20. Cooling Hibiscus Cooler:

**Ingredients:**

- 2 tbsp. hibiscus, dried
- 2 cups boiling water
- 1 lime's juice
- Optional: honey, sugar, and garnishes like orange slices or mint- Sliced oranges or mint leaves (for garnish)

**Instructions:**

- Place hibiscus in a teapot or infuser.
- Add hot water.
- Infuse for 10-15 mins.
- Filter, add lime juice, and sweeten if desired.
- Refrigerate and serve with garnish.

## 21. Mineral-Rich Nettle & Oat Straw Brew:

**Ingredients:**

- 1 tbsp. each of dried nettle and oat straw
- 2 cups hot water
- Optional: honey or lemon

**Instructions:**

- Combine nettle and oat straw in a teapot or infuser.
- Pour in boiling water.
- Let infuse for 15-20 mins.
- Strain, flavor if desired, and consume for its nutrients.

## 22. Warm Cinnamon Chai:

**Ingredients:**

- 1 cinnamon stick
- 2 black tea bags
- 4 cups boiling water
- 1 cup of any milk
- Optional: honey or sugar

**Instructions:**

- In a pot, combine cinnamon, tea bags, and hot water.
- Let sit for 5-7 mins.
- Add milk, warm for 5 more mins, then strain.
- Optionally sweeten and serve warmly.

## 23. Mineral-Rich Nettle & Oat Straw Brew:

**Ingredients:**

- 1 cup mint leaves
- 1/2 sliced cucumber
- 4 cups cold water
- 1 lemon's juice
- Optional: honey or sugar

**Instructions:**

- Mix mint and cucumber in a jug.
- Fill with water, add lemon juice, and sweeten if preferred.
- Refrigerate for 1 hour and serve cold.

## 24. Detoxifying Dandelion Tea:

**Ingredients:**

- 1 tbsp. dandelion root (dried)
- 1 cup boiling water
- Optional: honey or lemon

**Instructions:**

- Introduce dried dandelion to a teapot or infuser.
- Add the hot water.
- Allow it to sit for 5-10 mins.
- Filter, and optionally sweeten or flavor.
- Sip this brew for liver wellness.

## 25. Chamomile-Lemon Balm Calming Tea:

**Ingredients:**

- 1 tbsp. dried chamomile blossoms
- 1 tbsp. dried lemon balm
- 2 cups hot water
- Optional: honey

**Instructions:**

- Mix chamomile and lemon balm in a teapot or infuser.
- Introduce the boiling water.
- Infuse for 10-15 mins.
- Filter and sweeten if liked.
- Consume this blend for peace and alleviation of tension.

## 26. Anti-Inflammatory Turmeric Tea:

**Ingredients:**

- 1 tsp. turmeric powder
- 1/2 tsp. ginger powder
- 1/4 tsp. cinnamon powder
- A hint of black pepper
- 2 cups hot water
- Optional: honey or lemon

**Instructions:**

- Mix the turmeric, ginger, cinnamon, and pepper in a teapot or infuser.
- Add the boiling water to the spices.
- Allow a 5-10 minute steep time.
- Filter and optionally flavor or sweeten.
- Sip for its anti-inflammatory benefits.

## 27. Lemon Verbena and Echinacea Immunity Elixir:

**Ingredients:**

- 1 tbsp. dried echinacea
- 1 tbsp. dried lemon verbena
- 2 cups hot water
- Optional: honey or lemon

**Instructions:**

- Introduce echinacea and lemon verbena to a teapot or infuser.
- Pour boiling water over the mix.
- Infuse for 10-15 minutes.
- Filter, and sweeten or flavor if you like.
- Drink regularly for immune support..

## 28. Matcha Energy Boost:

**Ingredients:**

- 1 tsp. matcha powder
- 1 cup hot water (avoid boiling)
- Optional: honey or sugar

**Instructions:**

- Whisk the matcha in hot water until it's bubbly in a bowl.
- Add sweetness as per preference.
- Drink up and benefit from its antioxidants.

## 29. Relaxing Passionflower Infusion:

**Ingredients:**

- 1 tbsp. dried passionflower
- 1 cup boiling water
- Optional: honey or lemon

**Instructions:**

- Add the passionflower to a teapot or infuser.
- Introduce the boiling water.
- Allow 5-10 minutes of steeping.
- Filter, and add honey or lemon if you wish.
- Consume to foster relaxation and restful sleep.

## 30. Aromatic Jasmine Green Tea:

**Ingredients:**

- 1 tsp. jasmine green tea
- 1 cup hot water (avoid boiling)

**Instructions:**

- Place the jasmine tea in a teapot or infuser.
- Add the hot water.
- Steep for a brief 2-3 minutes.
- Filter and discard the used tea.
- Savor the fragrant taste of jasmine.

# Chapter 3: What to Use in Herbal Teas

The rich history of herbal teas spans centuries. Beyond their delightful taste, they offer numerous health benefits. Delve into the vast realm of herbal ingredients, unlocking the mysteries of their flavors and healing capacities.

## Unveiling Herbal Tea Components

**Popular Herbs:**

- Peppermint: Experience the refreshment of peppermint, noted for aiding digestion and enhancing mental sharpness.
- Chamomile: Relish the serene essence of chamomile, celebrated for promoting relaxation and deep sleep.
- Lemon Balm: Enjoy lemon balm's cheerful aura, a remedy for stress and a promoter of calm.
- Hibiscus: Taste the bold tanginess of hibiscus, lauded for its antioxidants and heart health benefits.
- Rosehips: Dive into rosehips' zesty taste, famous for their rich vitamin C and immune-boosting properties.

**Distinctive Ingredients:**

- Elderflower: Revel in the soft floral tones of elderflower, esteemed for bolstering immunity and clearing respiratory blockages.
- Rooibos: Relish rooibos' full-bodied flavors, a caffeine-less gem known to combat inflammation and nurture skin.
- Lavender: Submerge in lavender's soothing fragrance, aiding in stress reduction and better sleep.
- Ginger: Experience ginger's fiery taste, praised for digestive health and reducing inflammation.
- Turmeric: Feel the rustic essence of turmeric, acknowledged for combating inflammation and aiding joint health.

## Matching Ingredients with Health Benefits

**Digestive Health:**

- Peppermint & Ginger: Both renowned for soothing digestive ailments, from indigestion to nausea.
- Fennel: Acknowledged for easing digestion and reducing gas.

**Relaxation:**

- Chamomile, Lemon Balm & Lavender: All recognized for calming nerves and ensuring sound sleep.

**Immunity:**

- Echinacea, Elderflower & Rosehips: Champions of strengthening immune defenses.
- Astragalus: Promotes the production of white blood cells and overall immunity.

**Detox and Purification:**

- Dandelion: Recognized for supporting liver and digestion.
- Nettle: Helps in toxin removal and promotes clear skin.

## Mastering Herbal Tea Compositions

**Balancing Taste & Smell**:

- Learn to merge herbs for an ideal taste balance, such as coupling mild with robust herbs.
- Blend varied scents for an enriched herbal tea experience.

**Crafting Custom Mixes**:

- Experience the fun of crafting personal herbal mixes.
- Delve into tea energetics, aligning herbal energies with your own for harmony.

## Harvest, Preservation, and Tea Making Techniques

**Harvesting**:

- Understand the optimal harvest times for various herbs.
- Practice sustainable harvesting methods.

**Drying & Storing**:

- Familiarize yourself with herb preservation methods.
- Uncover strategies to keep dried herbs potent.

**Making Herbal Brews**:

- Master the craft of herbal tea making.
- Recognize the significance of proper steeping and temperatures.

Through understanding herbs' vast benefits, we can customize our teas to cater to health needs or relish in relaxation. Proper selection, blending, and brewing let us tap into the wonders of herbs, guiding us on a wellness and sensory journey. Whether for health or sheer enjoyment, herbal teas are a treasure for the soul, body, and mind.

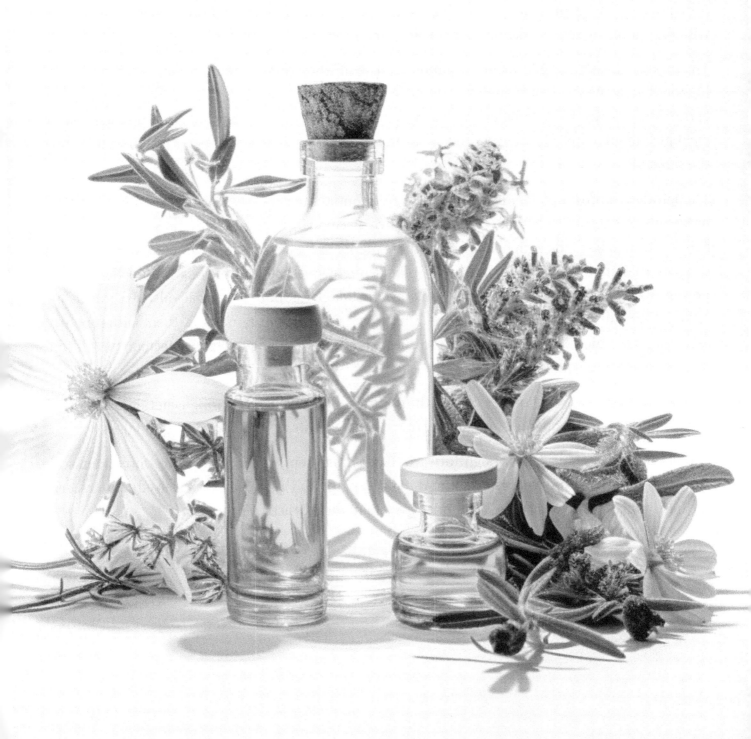

# BOOK 8: ESSENTIAL OILS

## Introduction

Essential oils, nature's potent elixirs, are derived from the various sections of plants, encompassing roots, seeds, flowers, barks, and more. These oils serve a dual purpose for plants: they act as protective agents against threats like harmful microbes and insects, and they also lure pollinators with their alluring scents, playing a vital role in the reproduction process.

The impact of essential oils is both profound and swift, showcasing their potency. Their strength is highlighted by the fact that even tiny amounts can have significant effects. Reflecting on the intricate extraction process, it's astonishing to learn that around 1.4 million hand-harvested rose blossoms yield just about a liter of rose essential oil, or that it takes sixty-seven roses for just a single drop of the same oil.

Though derived from plants, it's essential to differentiate between essential oils and other plant-based oils. For instance, oils like coconut and olive oil come from plant fruits and seeds. There's also a distinction to be made with infused oils, where plants like aloe vera are simmered in carrier oils to transfer their nutrients. And while some plants might need such infusions due to the minimal presence of essential oils, these shouldn't be mistaken for pure essential oils. Fragrance oils, although capturing the scent of plants, don't carry their benefits, making them different from essential oils. Think of essential oils as the encapsulation of a plant's defense mechanism, all while having an aromatic allure.

The spectrum of essential oils is vast, with offerings like Angelica root oil, asafetida oil, basil oil, bergamot oil, black pepper oil, and many others, each with its unique properties and uses.

Yet, obtaining these oils isn't straightforward. Extracting them, particularly on a commercial scale, demands expertise. The yield is often minimal compared to the raw materials used, underscoring the need for ensuring purity and minimizing waste in the extraction process.

# Chapter 1: Essential Oil

Essential oils truly capture the core essence of plants, justifying their "essential" label. They're derived from a special class of plant molecules called terpenes, or hydrocarbons, responsible for generating the distinct aromas of plants.

Terpenes serve as the plant's aromatic compounds, playing a critical role in their defense mechanism against pests. Many trees emit these aromatic terpenes, especially in hotter climates, which contribute to cloud formation, offering the tree a natural temperature regulation system. It's been established through studies that terpenes form the primary constituents of essential oils.

Every individual plant species boasts a distinct blend of over a hundred terpenes, resulting in their unique fragrances. These aromatic compounds can be located in various parts of a plant – be it the flowers, roots, leaves, stems, bark, or seeds. Beyond just lending their pleasant aromas, terpenes make these plants incredibly versatile. This versatility is reflected in their widespread applications, from being the fragrance in beauty and household items, to flavor enhancers in food, and even as therapeutic agents in various medicines.

Interestingly, though termed "essential oils", they aren't true oils in the traditional sense. Compare them with oils like canola, olive, almond, or sesame. When these oils are exposed to heat, such as during cooking, they retain their liquid state, earning them the title of fixed oils. Essential oils, on the other hand, vaporize when subjected to heat. This characteristic allows them to be readily inhaled in practices like aromatherapy, enhancing their medicinal value.

Fixed oils, whether sourced from plants or animals, typically encompass fatty acids. These fatty acids can play a pivotal role in ensuring dietary balance.

## What is Aromatherapy?

Aromatherapy is a holistic treatment strategy that leverages the healing properties of plant-derived essential oils to promote physical, mental, and emotional wellness. These oils are procured from plants using a method called distillation. With roots stretching back millennia, aromatherapy is a complementary medical practice built on the idea that certain plant aromas can profoundly impact our health and state of mind.

Essential oils are potent plant extracts that embody the plant's aromatic and intrinsic qualities. Techniques like steam distillation or cold pressing are employed to extract these oils, ensuring the preservation of the powerful compounds within.

Central to aromatherapy is the belief that inhaling or applying these oils can stimulate the brain's limbic system, a region governing various bodily functions, emotional responses, and associated memories. When breathed in or applied to the skin, essential oils can induce relaxation, mitigate stress, and foster bodily equilibrium, all owing to the oils' aromatic and chemical constituents.

**Popular aromatherapy methods encompass:**

- **Inhalation**: Essential oils can be diffused into the surrounding air using devices or directly inhaled from their container or a cloth. When inhaled, the aromatic molecules traverse the respiratory system, get absorbed into the bloodstream, and subsequently exert their influence on the body and psyche.
- **Topical** Use: By mixing essential oils with carriers like jojoba or almond oil, they can be applied to the skin either via massage or targeting specific regions. This topical application allows the oils to permeate the skin, rendering localized or broad benefits.
- **Bathing**: Incorporating several essential oil droplets into a warm bath results in a relaxing and fragrant escapade. As the oils blend with the water, they're absorbed via the skin, and their vapors inhaled.
- **Compresses**: This involves drenching a fabric in water mingled with essential oils and placing it onto a specific body part. Compresses can be therapeutic for pain mitigation, diminishing inflammation, or aiding wound recuperation.

The advantages of aromatherapy span stress relief, relaxation, better sleep quality, mood elevation, pain alleviation, immune fortification, and heightened attention and focus. Each essential oil offers distinct attributes, and blending various oils can amplify their combined effects.

Nonetheless, it's pivotal to understand that aromatherapy demands meticulous caution. Given the intense concentration of essential oils, it's paramount to dilute them aptly. Certain populations, like expectant mothers, infants, or those with particular health conditions, may need to sidestep some oils due to potential sensitivities or health implications. For a safe and beneficial aromatherapy experience, it's advisable to consult with a qualified aromatherapist or a healthcare professional.

## Essential Tools

In the realm of aromatherapy and essential oil use, certain instruments play pivotal roles in amplifying your experience, ensuring safety, and facilitating effective application. Here's an overview of the indispensable tools for an aromatherapy aficionado:

1. **Essential Oils**: At the heart of aromatherapy lies a selection of premium essential oils. Commence with versatile staples such as lavender, peppermint, tea tree, and lemon. Over time, tailor your collection to resonate with your unique preferences and requirements.

2. **Dark Glass Bottles**: Shield your essential oils from light degradation by storing them in tinted glass containers. Amber or cobalt blue hues are popular choices, equipped with secure lids or dropper functionalities. A spectrum of sizes will cater to diverse oil volumes.

3. **Carrier Oils**: To safely apply essential oils on the skin, they should be diluted using carrier oils. Top picks encompass sweet almond, jojoba, coconut, and grapeseed oils. Prioritize those that are cold-pressed, organic, and unrefined.

4. **Diffuser**: This device releases essential oil particles into the atmosphere, immersing you in their therapeutic fragrances. From ultrasonic and nebulizing to heat diffusers, pick one aligned with your needs.

5. **Personal Inhalers**: These compact devices permit direct essential oil inhalation. Tailored for mobility, they can be infused with bespoke oil concoctions targeting specific needs like relaxation or alleviating congestion.

6. **Massage Instruments**: For those who incorporate essential oils in massages, tools like massage rollers, bottles, or stones enhance the overall experience, ensuring uniform oil application and a tranquil massage session.

7. **Identification Aids**: Efficiently differentiate between your oils and blends with labels or markers. Opt for waterproof varieties to safeguard against fading or smearing.

8. **Literature and Digital Guides**: Enrich your understanding by investing in credible books or online platforms delving into essential oil nuances, blending techniques, and safety protocols.

9. **Protective Accessories**: Emphasize safety when mingling with essential oils. Stock up on disposable gloves, protective eyewear, and a shielding garment like a lab coat or apron, particularly if delving into concentrated concoctions.

10. **Knowledge Enhancement**: Beyond tangible tools, continuous learning is paramount. Engage in workshops, pursue courses, or seek mentorship from seasoned aromatherapists to refine your aromatherapy proficiency.

Always approach essential oils with respect, abide by suggested dosages and dilution rates, and ensure they're out of reach for young ones and pets. Equipped with these tools, you're poised to fully harness the restorative and calming potentials of essential oils.

## Extraction Methods

The diverse universe of essential oils is underpinned by the intricate methods employed to extract these aromatic elixirs. Here's a succinct exploration of the manifold extraction techniques:

1. **Distillation**: Dominating the industrial scene, distillation, notably steam distillation, reigns supreme. Here, plant matter is situated in expansive stainless steel containers. Injecting steam ruptures aroma-rich molecules, transitioning them into a gaseous state. This aromatic mist subsequently liquifies through a condenser. The complexity of this method necessitates specialized machinery and vigilant monitoring.

2. **Maceration**: Opting for carrier oils as solvents, maceration draws out aromatic properties from plants. A hallmark of macerated oils is their ability to encapsulate weightier plant constituents, yielding a denser aromatic footprint. This method's catch? It mandates exceedingly dry plant inputs.

3. **Enfleurage**: A nod to ancient extraction lore, enfleurage is seldomly adopted in contemporary times. This technique exists in two avatars: cold and hot, the latter introducing heat into the process. Vegetable fat forms the crux of this method, serving as a scent receptacle. Flowers or petals nestle into this fat, gradually infusing it with their aroma. To maximize potency, spent plant elements are substituted with fresh ones repeatedly. The aromatic crescendo is reached when the fat achieves saturation, after which alcohol intervenes, bifurcating the mix into essence-rich absolute and unfragranced fat.

4. **Cold Press/Expression**: Citrus fruits owe their aromatic extraction to this method. Dubbed expression or scarification, this technique punctures the citrus exterior, releasing sacs laden with essential oils. As these oils cascade out, mingling with other pigments, they are meticulously collected.

These intricate processes underscore an overarching truth: essential oils are therapeutic aromatic powerhouses. Their intrinsic fragrance sets them apart from generic oils. Recognizing this distinction is pivotal, especially when curating an essential oil collection or making a purchase. This aromatic essence not only captivates the senses but also offers myriad healing properties, rendering them indispensable in the realms of wellness and holistic care.

## The Components of Essential Oils

Essential oils are revered for their diverse aromatic properties and the range of therapeutic benefits they offer. These oils are essentially concentrated essences extracted from plants, and the unique chemical composition of each oil determines its scent, flavor, and therapeutic attributes.

Let's delve into the chemical maze of these oils:

1. **Aldehydes**: Best exemplified by lemongrass oil, aldehydes impart essential oils with antibacterial, anti-inflammatory, and antifungal characteristics. Oils abundant in aldehydes have a propensity to oxidize quickly, necessitating their replacement after roughly six

months. Given their potent nature, direct application to the skin is discouraged, with a recommended dilution of up to 1%.

2. **Lactones**: While they appear in a majority of essential oils, their concentration is often too trivial to be of significance. In excessive amounts, lactones may induce neurotoxic effects. However, given the minuscule amounts in essential oils, this concern is largely mitigated. One redeeming quality of lactones is their potential to combat respiratory infections.

3. **Esters**: Esters, predominant in oils such as mandarin and wintergreen, are credited for their sedative, antispasmodic, anti-inflammatory, and calming attributes. They are particularly adept at alleviating muscle tension and inflammation, making them ideal for those grappling with rheumatoid arthritis.

4. **Phenols**: Phenol-rich essential oils, like cinnamon, are potent antiseptics and disinfectants, boasting robust antibacterial and antimicrobial properties. However, they do come with their share of challenges; they can be harsh on the skin and taxing on the liver, prompting recommendations for short-term use.

5. **Ketones**: Treading into potentially treacherous territory, ketones, when abundant, can jeopardize the health of the liver and kidneys. Their use is advocated in strictly diluted form, with a concentration no greater than 1%. Yet, their capacity to assuage respiratory congestion cannot be dismissed, provided they're used judiciously.

6. **Terpenes**: Pervading almost all essential oils to varying extents, terpenes are especially profuse in citrus-based essential oils, accrediting these oils with their Vitamin C richness. Terpene-abundant oils serve as antimicrobial, anti-inflammatory, and antiviral agents. Moreover, they fortify the immune system and counteract diseases. Their antioxidant properties are instrumental in thwarting the deleterious effects of free radicals.

In the intricate tapestry of essential oils, each thread or compound has its distinct role and value. As with any potent substance, while the therapeutic benefits of essential oils are vast, prudence and informed usage are paramount. Whether you're using them for relaxation, therapeutic benefits, or their delightful aroma, understanding their chemistry can guide you to make the most of their myriad offerings.

# Chapter 2:    Herbs for Skin Beauty, Wellness and Health

## The Essence of Essential Oils

Essential oils are captivating in their aromatic allure and therapeutic capabilities. Extracted from plants, these oils encapsulate the volatile, aromatic substances housed within various parts of the plant, be it the leaves, roots, flowers, or even the resins and wood. Gazing deeper into the microscopic world of these plants, one finds tiny glands brimming with the essence that is transformed into essential oils.

### The Art of Extraction

Four predominant techniques grace the realm of essential oil extraction:

1. **Steam Distillation:** In this method, steam heats the plant material, liberating the essential oils, which are then condensed with water and separated.

2. **Expression**: During expression, oils are wrested either by centrifugation or by exerting pressure on the plant material.

3. **Solvent Extraction**: The plant material is bathed in a volatile solvent. As the solvent evaporates, it bequeaths behind a waxy substance termed 'concrete'. Distilling the concrete further yields the 'absolute', which is a potent concentration of the essential oil.

4. **Effleurage**: Though not elaborated in the initial explanation, effleurage involves pressing plant materials onto a fatty substance, allowing the aromatic compounds to infuse the fat.

It is crucial to discern that only those oils obtained without the use of chemicals can genuinely be classified as essential oils.

### The Healing Breath of Essential Oils

When introduced to our bodies, essential oils can find their way into our system in myriad ways. While some advocate the enhancement of absorption through heat or specific application points, scientific corroboration in this domain remains scant.

Inhalation of these oils can stir the limbic system, our brain's epicenter for emotions, behaviors, and memories. Thus, a mere whiff of a familiar aroma can transport us back to a cherished memory or a past emotion.

### The Essential Ten

While the pantheon of essential oils is vast, here's a succinct list of ten renowned ones:

- **Peppermint**: An invigorating oil that stimulates and aids digestion.

- **Lavender**: A tranquilizing herb renowned for stress alleviation.

- **Sandalwood**: A calming essence, bolstering concentration.

- **Bergamot**: Dual-action of stress relief and assuaging skin conditions.

- **Rose**: Uplifts spirits and combats anxiety.

- **Chamomile**: A mood-enhancing relaxant.

- **Ylang-Ylang**: Addresses headaches, skin woes, and nausea.

- **Tea Tree**: An immune-boosting, infection-fighting marvel.

- **Jasmine**: An antidote for depression and a childbirth aid.

- **Lemon**: A versatile oil addressing digestion, mood, and headaches.

**Legacy & Usage**

Historically, essential oils have been pillars of therapeutic practices. Modern extraction predominantly hinges on steam distillation, but bygone eras also witnessed cold pressing, ensuring premium oil quality.

When using essential oils for healing or pain relief, it's imperative to store them aptly, away from culinary elements. Direct application, using a cotton medium, is advisable, but it's paramount to employ pure, therapeutic-grade oils. Look for genuine labels that clearly state the therapeutic and medicinal nature of the product.

In the vast ocean of oils available, one must be vigilant. While many oils today bear the tag "natural", they are mere fragrances devoid of the therapeutic prowess of genuine essential oils. Such superficial oils not only lack medicinal potency but can also be potentially hazardous if ingested.

## Herbs for Skin

Throughout the ages, nature has equipped humanity with herbal remedies to combat a wide array of ailments. From minor aches to chronic diseases, these natural solutions have garnered the trust and attention of both traditional healers and modern science.

- **Aloe Vera**: Revered for its soothing properties, Aloe Vera's gel works wonders as a natural moisturizer and softener. Known to expedite wound healing, its innate constituents promote cellular regeneration and offer pain relief when applied topically.

- **Arnica**: A powerhouse of healing, the tropical preparations of Arnica flowers are unparalleled in curing wounds. It dons multiple hats - an analgesic, anti-inflammatory, and antiseptic. As highlighted by Dr. Day, it's an essential go-to post surgeries or trauma to diminish bruises and swelling. Recognizing its prowess, even the German government endorses Arnica for wound treatment.

- **Calendula**: Often known as the garden marigold, Calendula's blossoms have long been employed to address an array of skin concerns ranging from burns to rashes. For those struggling with hard-to-heal wounds or specific ulcers, this flower might just be their savior. Its versatility extends to calendula tea compresses and as a mouthwash to assuage oral soreness.

- **Comfrey**: Rooted in age-old traditions, Comfrey's leaves and roots act as catalysts in treating external injuries. They also double up as potent anti-inflammatories, ideal for thwarting rashes. However, a word of caution: its application is limited in duration and quantity due to potential toxicity concerns.

- **Tea Tree**: Indigenous to Asia and Australia, this towering evergreen has historically been the guardian against infections. From wartime antiseptics to contemporary solutions for skin woes, the extracted oil from tea tree leaves holds antimicrobial properties. Yet, remember, while it's a skin ally, it's an internal foe and should never be consumed.

- **Chamomile**: A panacea in its own right, Chamomile flowers have graced countless remedies. Be it a soothing tea for the stomach, an oral rinse for dental ailments, or a salve for skin troubles, its applications are diverse and reliable.

- **Cayenne**: Spicing up the realm of herbal remedies, Cayenne, especially its component capsaicin, promises anti-inflammatory and antibacterial benefits. Its mechanism revolves around depleting substance P from nerve endings, bestowing it with analgesic properties. While promising relief, initial applications might feel intense due to the release of substance-P.

Herbal remedies, while being nature's gift, come with their set of caveats. Dr. Day underscores the importance of being cognizant of potential allergies to any herbal constituents. If any skin condition persists or exacerbates, it's paramount to consult a medical professional. Always remember, nature offers solutions, but knowledge ensures their judicious use.

## Herbs for a Long Life

From the earliest civilizations to contemporary times, nature has graced humanity with an abundance of herbs, each harboring unique properties beneficial for both culinary and medicinal uses.

- **Ginseng**: Ginseng, or Ginnsuu as known in some regions, stands as a testament to heart health. By enhancing blood circulation, particularly under reduced oxygen scenarios, it ensures that the heart receives its vital share. Notably, it acts as a protective shield by mitigating blood platelet stickiness, significantly cutting down the threat of clot formation.

- **Cloves**: Revered across various herbal traditions, cloves bolster the digestive system with their inherent warming properties. Beyond that, they also play a pivotal role in supporting immune and respiratory systems, thanks to the presence of Eugenol essential oil. Not just a fragrant kitchen spice, cloves boast a high ORAC score, pointing to their antioxidant-rich nature. They also emerge as defenders against gastrointestinal intruders like parasites, fungi, and bacteria.

- **Garlic**: A cornerstone in herbal medicine, particularly in the East, garlic is more than just a kitchen staple. It wears multiple hats - be it managing cardiovascular markers, warding off a spectrum of infections, amplifying immune responses, or exhibiting antioxidant and antitumor properties. Truly, garlic's medicinal prowess is vast and varied.

- **Oregano**: A relative to several aromatic herbs, oregano packs a punch both as fresh leaves and as an essential oil. Remarkably, its antioxidant capacity even overshadows the revered blueberries! With its components like Beta-caryophyllene, it emerges as a potent anti-inflammatory agent.

- **Ginger**: Beyond being a culinary delight, ginger is renowned for housing compounds like Geraniol that counteract cancer. Its anti-inflammatory nature ensures heart health, proving effective in clot prevention. Furthermore, it stands as a bulwark against atherosclerosis while also fortifying the immune system.

- **Turmeric**: A golden spice with roots in Indian tradition, turmeric's power lies in curcumin. Known for its vibrant hue, this component offers a plethora of health benefits. From cutting heart attack risks substantially to rivaling the cardiovascular benefits of regular exercise, turmeric stands tall in its health-promoting properties. Besides, with curcumin in its arsenal, it's associated with brain protection, inflammation reduction, and even potential cancer treatments.

In sum, these herbs and spices underscore the symbiotic relationship between nature and human health. As they find their way into our dishes, they also weave into the fabric of our well-being, ensuring a life of vitality and vigor.

# Herbs for Wellness and Health

In the tapestry of holistic health, herbs and their derived essential oils have woven timeless tales of healing, rejuvenation, and serenity. These age-old botanical marvels have been the cornerstone for countless therapies, offering a natural antidote to many of today's ailments. Let's delve into their magic and learn how these can be an integral part of your wellness journey.

- **Lavender**: Lavender, often described as nature's tranquilizer, is not just a visual treat but a therapeutic boon. It's not only about its visually captivating purple blossoms but the essence it encapsulates. With an array of applications from a diffuser, bathwater to massages, it's the go-to for mental relaxation and skin comfort.

- **Peppermint**: This zesty herb is a powerhouse of refreshment and rejuvenation. Apart from its aromatic presence in kitchens, its essential oil stands as a testament to vitality - be it in aiding digestion, breathing life into tired minds, or offering respite from headaches.

- **Eucalyptus**: Standing tall and permeating a distinct invigorating aroma, eucalyptus is a guardian of respiratory health. With versatile uses spanning from air purification, steam inhalation, to massages, it's nature's answer to clear breathing and muscular relief.

- **Rosemary**: Rosemary's robust herbal scent is not just a culinary delight. It transcends kitchens to infuse energy, stimulate memory, and ensure hair health. Whether you wish for mental agility, lustrous hair, or a circulatory boost, rosemary has got you covered.

- **Chamomile**: A symbol of gentleness, chamomile is the silent whisperer of peace. Whether it's about paving the way for restful sleep, soothing aggravated skin, or ensuring digestive comfort, chamomile, with its sweet notes, embraces you in its calming fold.

In Essence: At the heart of essential oils lie these magnificent herbs. Each, in its unique way, sings praises of nature's therapeutic genius. Whether you're seeking relaxation with lavender, invigoration with peppermint, clear breathing with eucalyptus, mental rejuvenation with rosemary, or sheer calmness with chamomile - nature has a solution.

Embark on this aromatic journey and let these essential oils guide your path to holistic health. In each drop, you'll discover nature's essence, ready to balance and nurture every facet of your being, ensuring a life brimming with well-being and harmony.

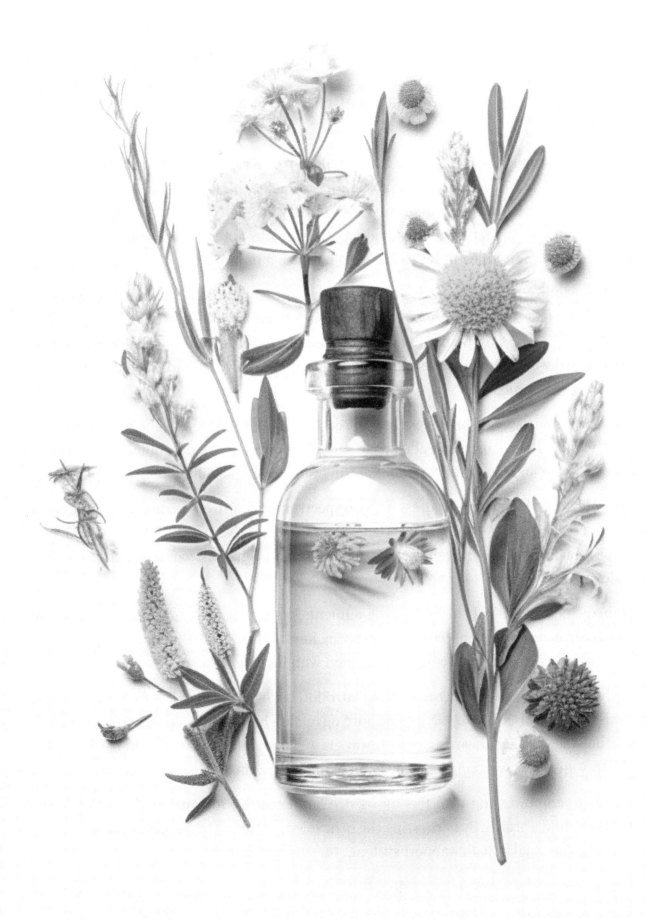

# BOOK 9: HERBAL MEDICINE FOR CHILDREN

## Introduction

Welcome to the enchanting world of holistic health tailored for our younger generation. This guide offers a deep dive into the herbal realm, spotlighting remedies that have been cherished over millennia to ensure the well-being of children. As we journey through these pages, we'll familiarize ourselves with a myriad of herbs, understanding their gentle potency in remedying common childhood ailments, from soothing upset tummies to bolstering immunity.

Our chief responsibility as guardians is to ensure the optimal health of our young ones. By harnessing the healing essence of plants, herbal medicine extends a well-tested avenue to bolster their overall health, addressing pediatric concerns while enhancing vitality. This volume melds time-honored herbal wisdom with modern insights, equipping you with a thorough understanding of child-friendly herbal remedies.

Our exploration commences with an insight into the core tenets of herbal medicine, elucidating how these natural wonders can complement a child's health journey. We'll spotlight the nuanced strength of these herbs and the significance of tailoring remedies to a child's specific needs.

Navigating through the chapters, we address a broad spectrum of health concerns, suggesting herbal solutions for everything from minor sniffles and fevers to digestive woes and skin complaints. Essential topics such as dosages, application methods, and when to consult experts will be thoroughly detailed.

Yet, herbal medicine isn't just about addressing ailments. Its essence lies in proactive care. We'll delve into preventive measures, emphasizing bolstering immunity and championing overall growth and development using herbal interventions combined with healthy habits.

A recurrent theme in our guide is the responsible introduction of herbs to children. We touch upon frequently raised questions, offering advice on sourcing quality herbs, concocting remedies, and the imperative of liaising with healthcare experts. Always remember, herbal treatments are meant to be a complementary approach, working hand-in-hand with modern medicine.

This guide aims to empower you with the knowledge and expertise to confidently employ herbal remedies for your child's health. By harnessing the benevolent nature of herbs, you're poised to offer them a nurturing, safe, and holistic support system.

May this book serve as a trusty companion in your herbal journey. Let it kindle a deeper bond with Mother Nature and her verdant offerings. Together, let's walk the path of holistic wellness, leaning on the age-old wisdom of herbal remedies to foster the well-being of our precious young ones.

# Chapter 1: 0-2 Months

**The Delicate Nature of Newborns**

The first two months of an infant's life are crucial for adapting to life outside the womb. During this time, their bodies undergo rapid changes, and they face unique health challenges. In this chapter, we will delve deeper into common health issues and how certain herbal remedies can offer relief, always emphasizing the utmost caution and consultation with healthcare professionals.

**Common Health Issues for Newborns**

1. **Colic:** Often presenting in the first few weeks of life, colic is characterized by frequent and intense crying spells that aren't easily comforted. While its exact cause is uncertain, digestive discomfort is frequently suspected.

2. **Diaper Rash:** This is a common inflammation of the skin in the diaper area. Factors like wet diapers, friction, and skin sensitivity can contribute to diaper rash.

3. **Cradle Cap:** This condition manifests as yellowish, crusty patches on a baby's scalp and is caused by the excessive production of sebum.

**Herbal Remedies and Specific Recipes for Newborns**

1. **Chamomile for Colic Relief**

*Recipe: Chamomile Tea*

**Ingredients:**

- 1/2 teaspoon dried chamomile flowers
- 8 oz boiling water

**Instructions:**

- Boil the water and remove from heat.
- Add the chamomile flowers.
- Cover and steep for 5 minutes.
- Strain the tea to remove all the chamomile flowers.

- Allow to cool to room temperature before giving to the baby.

*Usage:* Consult with a pediatrician for the appropriate amount to give. Generally, 1-2 teaspoons can be offered, but always start with the smallest amount.

2. **Calendula for Diaper Rash**

*Recipe: Calendula Oil*

## Ingredients:

- 1 cup of calendula flowers (dried)
- 2 cups of a carrier oil (like olive oil or almond oil)

## Instructions:

- Place calendula flowers in a jar.
- Pour the carrier oil over the flowers until they are fully submerged.
- Seal the jar and place it in a sunny spot for 4-6 weeks.
- Strain the oil to remove the flowers and store in a cool, dark place.
- *Usage:* Apply a small amount of the oil to the affected area after each diaper change.

## Dosage and Preparation Methods

Always ensure herbs are pure and organic, especially when intended for newborns. When preparing remedies, sterilize all utensils and storage containers. Start with the smallest suggested dose and monitor for any reactions. If any adverse reactions occur, discontinue use and consult a healthcare provider immediately.

## Cautions and Potential Side Effects

Herbs, though natural, can still have potent effects on a newborn's body. Always monitor for allergic reactions after introducing a new remedy. Signs of an allergic reaction can include redness, swelling, rash, or unusual fussiness. If any of these signs present, cease use and seek medical advice immediately.

# Chapter 2: 2-12 Months

Herbal medicine capitalizes on the therapeutic qualities of plants and is viewed as an alternative and complementary medical option. However, special care should be taken when considering these remedies for young ones, particularly those aged 2-12 months. Infants, with their sensitive systems, may have different reactions to these herbs than older kids or adults do. Always seek advice from a pediatrician or healthcare specialist before giving children any herbal treatments. Here are some herbs often suggested for babies:

1. **Chamomile**:

Recognized for its gentle nature, chamomile can address digestive problems like colic and can have a calming effect, possibly leading to improved sleep. While small amounts of chamomile tea can be given to babies, proper dilution and quantity is crucial. For chamomile tea:

- Pour boiling water over a teaspoon of dried chamomile flowers.
- Allow it to infuse for 5-10 minutes.
- After straining the tea, cool it down.
- Ensure the tea is suitably diluted before giving it to the baby.

2. **Fennel**:

Fennel seeds have gained a reputation for alleviating digestive issues in babies like gas and indigestion. To prepare fennel tea:

- Add some crushed fennel seeds to hot water.
- Allow the tea to brew for 5-10 minutes.
- After straining the tea, cool it down.
- As with chamomile, make sure the tea is properly diluted for babies.

3. **Ginger**:

Traditionally, ginger has been a remedy for digestive problems and nausea. It might be useful for babies with mild stomach issues. For ginger tea:

- Place a tiny slice of fresh ginger into boiling water.
- Let it brew for 5-10 minutes.

- After straining, allow the tea to cool.
- Remember to be cautious with ginger and keep the amount minimal to prevent possible side effects.

4. **Echinacea**:

It's worth noting that Echinacea isn't typically advised for infants due to insufficient evidence and potential risks. Always consult with a healthcare expert before even thinking about Echinacea for babies.

5. **Calendula**:

Frequently known as marigold, calendula is typically used on the skin to address issues like diaper rashes or minor cuts. After getting a nod from a healthcare expert, calendula-based creams with few ingredients can be used on babies. For application:

- Clean the problem area with mild soap and warm water.
- Dry the skin with a soft cloth.
- Take a small amount of the calendula product.
- Apply it to the problem area with gentle, circular motions.
- This can be repeated 2-3 times daily or based on healthcare advice.

Emphasizing again, using herbal solutions for infants should always be under the supervision of a medical expert who can offer tailored advice for the child's specific health scenario. Ensure the treatments are safe, apt, and administered correctly. Furthermore, always keep in mind that not every herb is baby-friendly, and some might even be dangerous. Babies have unique dosage needs, and the potency of herbal products should be evaluated meticulously. Always approach herbal treatments for infants with caution, backed by proper research and professional guidance.

# Chapter 3: 12 Months – 5 Years

Using herbal medicine as a supplementary method to bolster health and wellness is possible for children between 12 months and 5 years of age. Nonetheless, it's vital to recognize that the systems of children within this age bracket are still maturing. Therefore, one must be prudent when considering herbs. Before incorporating any herbal treatments for youngsters, a conversation with a pediatrician or health expert is imperative.

Outlined below are a few herbal solutions frequently recommended for children between 12 months and 5 years:

1. **Elderberry**:

Recognized for its capacity to fortify the immune system, elderberry can assist in minimizing the intensity and length of symptoms associated with colds and flu. Syrups or gummies made from elderberry, designed especially for kids, can be found in several health-focused stores. When giving elderberry-based products to kids:

- Abide by the dosage guidelines on the product's label.
- Confirm that products are child-centric and devoid of allergens or detrimental additives.
- Provide the correct dose, keeping the child's age and weight in mind, as advised by health experts.

2. **Peppermint**:

Often chosen for addressing digestive discomforts like stomach pains and bloating, peppermint tea can be offered to children older than 2 years but in controlled amounts. However, it's not suitable for very young kids because of potential breathing issues. For making peppermint tea for children:

- Infuse a teaspoon of dried peppermint in boiling water.
- Allow it to settle for around 5-10 minutes.
- Filter the tea and cool it down.
- Serve it to children, ensuring it's at a comfortable temperature.

3. **Lemon Balm**:

This soothing herb can aid in reducing stress and enhancing relaxation and sleep. You can find it as herbal teas or as essential oils for aromatic use. For using the oil:

- Mix a few drops of lemon balm oil with carrier oils like almond or coconut.
- Apply this mix gently onto areas like the child's temples to induce relaxation and sleep.

- Alternatively, lemon balm tea can be brewed and given to the child following the peppermint tea guidelines.

4. **Licorice Root**:

With properties that provide relief from cough and throat irritation, you can find licorice root in cough syrups made for children. Given its potential side effects, ensure it's used judiciously and for short periods. For licorice root syrups:

- Stick to the dosage mentioned on the product.
- Opt for syrups created especially for children, ensuring they lack harmful ingredients.
- Dispense the right dose, based on a pediatrician's guidance.

5. **Eucalyptus**:

Proper usage of eucalyptus oil can help alleviate symptoms of respiratory infections. However, avoid using it around infants. For children, consider diffusing the oil in their rooms. For this:

- Follow the user manual for filling vaporizers or diffusers.
- Introduce a couple of eucalyptus oil drops.
- Ensure the device is safely positioned away from the child's access.

6. **Ginger**:

Beneficial for digestive issues, ginger can be served as tea or through ginger-rich foods to children over 2 years. For ginger tea:

- Start by slicing fresh ginger after peeling.
- Immerse these slices in boiling water.
- Allow it to steep for a while, then strain and cool.
- Provide the tea to children, making sure it's not too warm.

Always be mindful of the distinctive sensitivities kids might have towards herbal solutions. Before diving into herbal treatments, consulting with healthcare professionals is essential. They can provide insights regarding doses, potential drug interactions, and the suitability of herbs based on the child's health. Lastly, sourcing herbal products from trusted establishments that prioritize child safety and quality is of the utmost importance.

# Chapter 4: Herbal Remedies for Children Aged 5 to 12 Years

In considering herbal treatments for kids between 5 and 12 years, one must recognize that their bodies are still maturing and might react differently to herbs than adults do. It's always vital to seek advice from a pediatrician or medical expert before giving any herbal products to children of this age bracket. These experts can offer guidance tailored to a child's unique health needs and conditions.

Below is a list of frequently used herbal solutions for kids within the 5 to 12 age range:

### 1. Echinacea (Echinacea purpurea)

Commonly employed to reinforce the immune system, echinacea can be a powerful tool against cold symptoms. It's imperative to choose products that are age-appropriate for children and to follow dosage advice from health or herbal specialists. Echinacea may not be suitable for children with autoimmune conditions or those with allergies to plants like daisies.

How to Use:

- Echinacea tea: Combine 1 teaspoon of dried echinacea with a cup of boiling water for 10 minutes. Strain and let it cool before giving 1-2 teaspoons to the child three times daily for up to 10 days to aid against colds or respiratory infections.

- Echinacea syrup: Mix a teaspoon of dried echinacea root with a cup of water in a saucepan. Simmer for 15 minutes, strain, then add a cup of honey and continue to simmer for an additional 10 minutes. Store in a glass bottle. Give 1 teaspoon to the child 2-3 times daily during illness to boost immunity.

### 2. Chamomile (Matricaria chamomilla)

Chamomile is renowned for its tranquilizing qualities, aiding in digestive problems, restlessness, and slight anxiety. For the young ones, a diluted chamomile beverage can be prepared using a minor quantity of dried chamomile. Ensure it's adequately cooled before administration and adjust as per a healthcare expert's guidance. Usage:

- Chamomile tea: Allow 1 teaspoon of dried chamomile to sit in 1 cup of hot water for 5 minutes. Strain, cool, and serve 1/4 to 1/2 cup to the child 2-3 times daily to encourage relaxation, better sleep, or address digestive troubles.

- Chamomile bath: Secure a handful of dried chamomile in a cloth bag and place it under the tap during a child's bath. A 10-15 minute soak in this infusion can be relaxing and beneficial for skin issues.

### 3. Lemon Balm (Melissa officinalis)

Celebrated for its soothing effects, lemon balm can assist with anxiety, restlessness, and sleep issues. Tea can be made using dried leaves of this herb. It's wise to start with a minimal quantity and modify strength based on the child's requirements and age. Always seek advice from a qualified professional regarding dosages. Usage:

- Lemon balm tea: Immerse 1 teaspoon of dried lemon balm in 1 cup of hot water for 5 minutes. After straining and cooling, give 1/4 to 1/2 cup to your child 2-3 times daily for issues like anxiety or restlessness.

- Lemon balm oil: Combine 1 teaspoon of dried lemon balm with 1/2 cup of a carrier oil (e.g., almond or olive). Shake daily and let it infuse for 2 weeks. After straining, apply a bit to the child's temples or wrists at bedtime for relaxation.

### 4. Peppermint (Mentha piperita)

Peppermint can offer relief from digestive discomforts like gas, bloating, and minor stomach pains. However, it's not recommended for kids below five due to possible risks like triggering reflux or hindering iron absorption. For older children, a mild peppermint tea can be made. Always get advice from a health expert regarding usage. Usage:

- Peppermint tea: Let 1 teaspoon of dried peppermint leaves sit in 1 cup of hot water for 5 minutes. After straining and cooling, administer 1/4 to 1/2 cup to your child 2-3 times daily for digestive relief.

- Peppermint oil rub: Mix a few drops of peppermint essential oil with a carrier oil. Gently rub a small amount on the child's stomach in circular motions for relief.

### 5. Valerian (Valeriana officinalis)

Commonly employed for relaxation and better sleep, valerian is typically not suggested for children under 12 unless supervised by a professional. Valerian can be consumed as tea, tinctures, or capsules. Always follow guidance from a healthcare or herbal expert regarding dosages. Usage:

- Valerian tea: Allow 1 teaspoon of dried valerian root to immerse in 1 cup of hot water for 10 minutes. Strain, cool, and provide 1/4 to 1/2 cup to the child 30 minutes before sleep for relaxation.

- Valerian tincture: For valerian tincture, it's best to get direction from an experienced herbalist.

### 6. Ginger (Zingiber officinale)

Ginger is esteemed for aiding digestion and can reduce nausea and stomach discomfort. For older kids, a tea made from fresh ginger root can be beneficial. You can also sweeten it mildly with honey. As always, seek advice from a healthcare professional regarding dosages. Usage:

- Ginger tea: Steep a slice of fresh ginger root in 1 cup of hot water for 10 minutes. After straining and cooling, serve 1/4 to 1/2 cup to your child for digestive relief.

- Ginger candies: Opt for naturally made ginger candies or chews, giving them sparingly to the child for relief from nausea or motion sickness.

### 7. Elderberry (Sambucus nigra)

Famous for its immune-enhancing capabilities, elderberry is often employed against cold and flu symptoms. Note that raw or immature elderberries can be harmful. Always opt for commercially made products or guidance from an herbal expert. Usage:

- Elderberry syrup: Adhere to the instructions on commercial elderberry syrups for dosing and usage. It can be a great aid for cold and flu symptoms, but always consult a professional for advice.

### 8. Calendula (Calendula officinalis)

Calendula is appreciated for its calming and anti-inflammatory qualities, making it a go-to for skin issues like rashes or minor wounds. It's best applied externally as creams or infused oils. Before full use, conduct a patch test to rule out allergies. Always rely on a professional's guidance for dosages and application. Usage:

- Calendula cream: Apply a layer of calendula cream on affected skin areas. Adhere to the product's instructions or seek guidance from a healthcare expert.

### 9. Marshmallow Root (Althaea officinalis)

Marshmallow root is favored for alleviating sore throats and coughs. A tea can be made by steeping the dried root in hot water. Once cooled, it can be given to the child. Additionally, a natural cough syrup can be prepared with guidance from an expert. Consultation with a healthcare professional is essential for proper dosage. Usage:

- Marshmallow root tea: Let 1 teaspoon of dried root steep in 1 cup of hot water for 10 minutes. Strain, cool, and offer 1/4 to 1/2 cup to the child up to three times daily for relief.

- Marshmallow root syrup: Rely on an expert herbalist's guidance for dosage and preparation of this syrup.

### 10.      Catnip (Nepeta cataria)

Catnip, recognized for its tranquilizing qualities, can be employed to mitigate restlessness or minor anxiety in children. A mild tea made from the dried leaves can be beneficial. Adjust strength based on the child's requirements and age, and always consult with a healthcare expert. Usage:

- Catnip tea: Steep 1 teaspoon of dried catnip leaves in 1 cup of hot water for 5 minutes. After straining and cooling, administer 1/4 to 1/2 cup to the child 1-2 times daily for relaxation.

## 11. Lemon Verbena (Aloysia citrodora)

Esteemed for its digestive relief properties, lemon verbena can be a wonderful aid for digestive discomforts in children. A tea made from dried leaves can be provided. As always, the strength and dose should be adjusted based on the child's age and health conditions, consulting with an expert when needed. Usage:

- Lemon verbena tea: Allow 1 teaspoon of dried leaves to immerse in 1 cup of hot water for 5-10 minutes. After straining and cooling, serve 1/4 to 1/2 cup to your child up to three times daily for digestive relief.

## 12. Licorice (Glycyrrhiza glabra)

Licorice is known for its soothing capabilities, especially for the throat and to reduce coughing. Yet, it should be used with caution due to potential side effects. Always employ under supervision and for limited durations. Consultation with a healthcare expert is a must before giving licorice to children. Usage:

- Licorice tea: Giving licorice tea to children requires guidance from a health specialist. If approved, prepare it following professional instructions and monitor the child's response carefully. It should be given in limited amounts and for short periods.

Always make sure to seek advice from healthcare experts or herbal specialists for detailed recommendations on dosage, application, and safety measures when considering herbal treatments for kids. Moreover, keep your healthcare practitioner informed about any medicines or supplements your child might be using to prevent possible interactions.

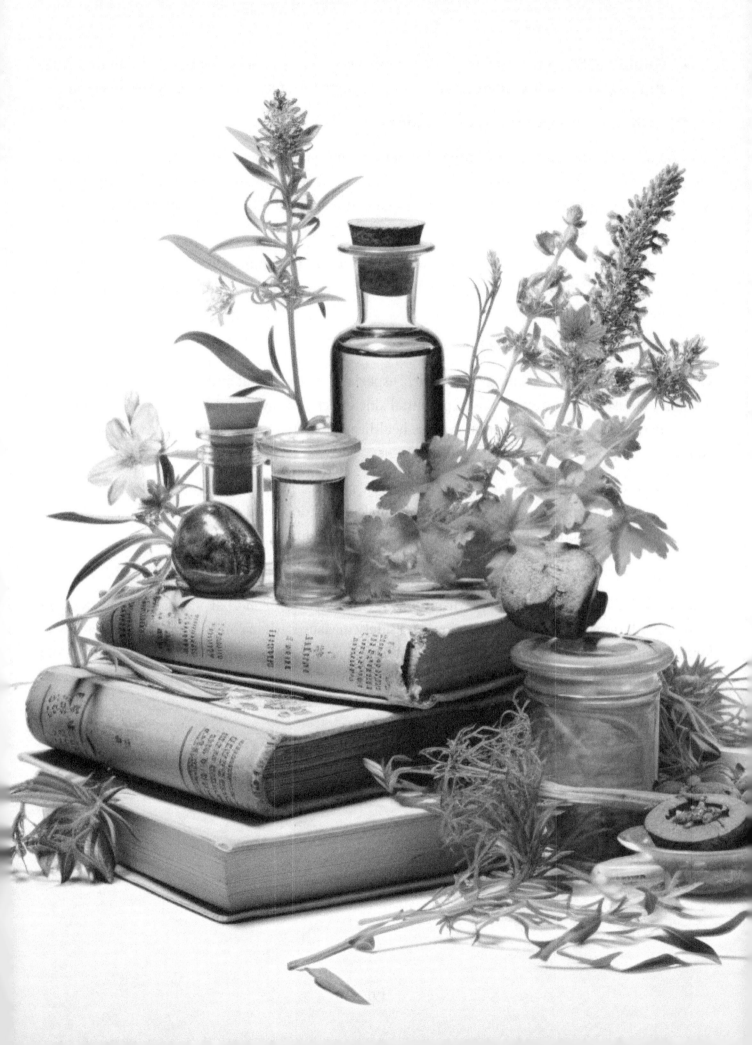

# BOOK 10:  FAQ

## How can one identify and find edible wild plants?

To spot and find wild plants that are safe to eat, one must blend their understanding with meticulous observation. Educate yourself on plant identification by delving into field guides or joining foraging expeditions guided by a seasoned expert. It's essential to be adept at noticing distinct characteristics like leaf shapes, flower designs, and typical habitats. Get acquainted with the local natural habitats around you and continuously expand your expertise. Before consuming any plant, always ensure its identity, as some edible plants have toxic look-alikes.

## What's the process for cleaning harvested herbs?

Properly cleaning harvested herbs is vital to remove unwanted pests, soil, or other impurities. Start by lightly shaking the herbs to dislodge any loose dirt, and then inspect for bugs or damaged sections. Wash the herbs under running lukewarm water or immerse them briefly in a basin. By gently moving the herbs with your hands, ensure all dirt is removed. If the herbs are delicate, dry them using a salad spinner or pat them with a clean cloth. Handle the herbs gently to prevent any damage. Once cleaned, store them appropriately for future use.

## How did Native Americans discern the medicinal properties of plants?

Over several generations, Native Americans deciphered the medicinal attributes of plants using observation, trial-and-error, and the verbal exchange of knowledge. They studied nature in-depth, concentrating on how plants interacted with their environment. This knowledge, achieved through hands-on experiences, instincts, and community interactions, was shared across generations via oral storytelling, ceremonies, and mentorships, preserving the invaluable wisdom about medicinal herbs.

## Why did Native Americans resort to medicinal herbs and what did they believe?

Medicinal herbs were integral to Native American traditions for multiple reasons. They recognized the interconnectedness of all life forms, viewing plants as sacred allies in maintaining both physical and spiritual balance. They employed herbs to address various ailments, encompassing physical, mental, and spiritual dimensions. They believed that plants possessed unique energies, like enhancing stamina, aiding childbirth, promoting vigor, or shielding from negative forces. Their comprehensive approach to wellness integrated the use of medicinal herbs.

## How can you ascertain if a herb is dry?

To verify a herb's dryness, its moisture level must be examined. Generally, a dry herb feels brittle, lacks moisture, and crumbles easily. It shouldn't feel moist or soft. Visually inspect the herb for dried and faded leaves and stems. For precise results, employ tools like a food dehydrator, a low-temperature oven, or air drying techniques. Properly dried herbs can be stored for longer durations without the threat of mold or decay.

## What does plant edibility testing entail, and how do you conduct it?

Plant edibility testing is a systematic approach to determine a plant's safety for consumption. After properly identifying the plant, begin by rubbing a fragment of it on your skin to check for allergic reactions. If safe, proceed by placing a minute quantity on your lips and observe for any discomfort or adverse reactions. Finally, place a tiny bit on your tongue and monitor for unusual tastes or feelings. It's imperative to approach plant edibility with caution and, when feasible, consult a professional forager or herbalist. Thorough understanding and caution are essential when foraging, as some plants might harbor toxic elements or demand particular preparation techniques for safe consumption.

## What herbs are typically used for stress and anxiety relief?
Several herbs are known to alleviate stress and anxiety, such as:

- **Chamomile**: Recognized for its soothing effects, chamomile aids in relaxation and reducing anxiety.
- **Lavender**: With its tranquilizing aroma, lavender aids in stress and anxiety reduction.
- **Valerian root**: This root is a natural choice for easing anxiety and tackling sleep issues.
- **Ashwagandha**: An adaptogenic herb, ashwagandha helps the body cope with stress and instills a calming sensation.
- **Lemon balm**: This herb is renowned for inducing relaxation and mitigating anxiety.

## Which herbal treatments assist with insomnia and enhance sleep?
Certain herbs can address insomnia and foster improved sleep:

- **Valerian root**: Renowned as a natural sleep enhancer, it can bolster sleep quality.
- **Passionflower**: With its sedative attributes, passionflower aids in sleep induction and boosts sleep quality.
- **Lavender**: Its serene scent fosters relaxation and sleep.
- **Chamomile**: Drinking chamomile tea can combat sleep disturbances.

- **Lemon balm**: This herb can diminish anxiety and foster improved sleep.

## Can herbal solutions address digestive problems like bloating or indigestion?

Yes, some herbs can combat digestive ailments like bloating and indigestion:

- **Peppermint**: Whether as oil or tea, peppermint can relax gastrointestinal tract muscles and ease bloating and indigestion.
- **Ginger**: Valued for its digestive benefits, ginger can mitigate bloating and foster digestion.
- **Fennel**: Consuming fennel seeds or tea can ease gas, bloating, and indigestion.
- **Chamomile**: Drinking chamomile tea can calm the digestive system and alleviate bloating and indigestion.

## What herbs have traditionally fortified the immune system?

Certain herbs have traditionally been used to bolster immunity:

- **Echinacea**: Widely utilized to boost immunity, it can diminish the duration and intensity of colds and flu.
- **Astragalus**: This herb fortifies the immune system and enhances defense mechanisms.
- **Elderberry**: Packed with antioxidants, elderberry has immune-boosting properties, particularly for respiratory infections.
- **Garlic**: Its antimicrobial and immune-boosting attributes can bolster immunity.
- **Ginseng**: As an adaptogenic herb, ginseng can modulate immune responses and bolster overall immunity.

## How can herbal solutions promote women's health, like menstrual pain or menopausal symptoms?

Herbs can be harnessed to address women's health issues:

- **Menstrual cramps**: Ginger, cinnamon, and cramp bark are known to ease pain and inflammation.
- **Menopause**: Black cohosh and dong quai can tackle menopausal symptoms like hot flashes.
- **Pregnancy**: Red raspberry leaf tea is used to fortify the uterus during pregnancy.
- **Hormonal imbalances**: Vitex or chasteberry can stabilize menstrual cycles and ease PMS.
- **Mood changes**: St. John's wort can address mood shifts and mild depression related to hormonal fluctuations.

## What natural solutions can treat skin conditions like acne or eczema?

For skin ailments, some natural remedies are:

- **Tea tree oil**: Its antibacterial properties can help diminish acne.
- **Aloe vera**: Beneficial for conditions like eczema, aloe vera gel can pacify skin and accelerate healing.
- **Calendula**: Applied topically, it can soothe eczema symptoms.
- **Witch hazel**: Its astringent properties can help manage acne.
- **Chamomile**: Beneficial for multiple skin irritations, including acne and eczema.

## Which herbs offer natural pain relief for ailments like headaches or muscle discomfort?

Certain herbs offer natural pain relief:

- **Willow bark**: Containing salicin, akin to aspirin, it can ease pain.
- **Ginger**: With its anti-inflammatory benefits, ginger can alleviate headache and muscle pain.
- **Peppermint**: It can relax muscles and alleviate tension headaches.
- **Turmeric**: Containing curcumin, it has anti-inflammatory properties.
- **Eucalyptus**: Used topically, it can diminish muscle discomfort.

## Can herbs assist with respiratory wellness and alleviate cold and allergy symptoms?

Absolutely, various herbs can boost respiratory health and mitigate symptoms associated with colds and allergies. For instance:

- **Echinacea:** This herb bolsters the immune system, potentially decreasing cold symptoms' intensity and length.
- **Peppermint:** Its properties can help decongest and relieve symptoms like nasal blockage and cold-induced coughs.
- **Ginger:** It has the potential to counter inflammation in respiratory passages and ease allergies and related infections.
- **Nettle leaf:** This leaf is beneficial for counteracting allergic reactions such as itchiness and sneezing.
- **Licorice root:** Beneficial for calming sore throats and reducing coughs and congestion.

## Are there risks when pairing herbal solutions with prescribed drugs?

Indeed, combining herbal treatments with prescription drugs requires caution. Herbs can interact with medicines and cause complications. Therefore, it's essential to:

- Discuss with a medical expert before introducing herbs to your medication regime.
- Be aware of possible herb-drug interactions.

- Always inform your doctor about any herbs or medications you're on.
- Adhere to dosage recommendations and monitor for unexpected reactions.
- When unsure, seek advice from an expert in herbal treatments.

## How can one integrate herbal treatments daily for improved health?

For a holistic health approach using herbs:

- Seek advice from an herbal specialist to identify the most suitable herbs for your needs.
- Invest time in understanding the right use, dosage, and method of each herb.
- Add herbs to your daily regimen through teas, tinctures, or other recommended forms.
- Stay consistent and adjust as required based on your body's feedback.

## How do standardized herbal extracts differ from whole herb formulations?

They differ in content and how they're produced:

- Standardized extracts emphasize certain active components, ensuring consistent strength.
- Whole herb methods employ the complete plant, retaining its natural constituents, and can be used in various forms.

## Is it safe to consume herbs during pregnancy and lactation?

Herb usage during pregnancy and nursing needs prudence:

- Always consult with an expert on herbal medicine beforehand.
- Some herbs might pose risks for the mother or fetus.
- Even commonly known herbs might be unsuitable during these phases.
- Ensure herbs chosen are based on thorough research and individual conditions.

## What are adaptogens, and how do they impact the body's reaction to stress?

Adaptogens, a category of herbs, aid the body in better handling stress:

- Herbs like ashwagandha and ginseng modulate stress hormones and fortify the adrenal glands.
- They elevate stamina, heighten resilience, and support overall health.
- Adaptogens also aid systems impacted by prolonged stress, such as immunity.
- Continuous consumption can maximize their positive impact on stress resilience.

## Can there be interactions between herbal treatments and other natural products?

Certainly, herbs might interact with other supplements or natural remedies. Hence:

- Combining certain herbs can lead to intense effects or unwanted reactions.
- It's wise to get advice from experts familiar with herb compatibility.
- Reveal all existing medications and health issues when considering herbal treatments.

In summary, while herbs offer substantial health benefits, their usage should be informed, careful, and under professional guidance.

Made in the USA
Las Vegas, NV
22 October 2023

79506429R00109